# Beyond Survival Tactics

## Life and Career Sustainability
for
Peace Officers

**John R. Engbeck, Editor**
**Terry Anderson**
**Stacey Forges**
**James E. Konopasek**
**J. E. Ruesch**
**Harold R. Torrens**

**Foreword by Commander Michael J. Nila**

**RivenDell Productions**
Box 536
Garden Valley, California
95633

# Acknowledgements

The authors express heartfelt gratitude for the thoughtful attention given to this work by colleagues and cohorts throughout the country. Likewise, we are grateful to the academic researchers in criminology, medicine, psychology, philosophy and theology, with special appreciation for Dr. John Violanti's research and dedication to police-officer health. And of course, we are grateful to the peace officers whose health and well-being are the subject of this work.

**John R. Engbeck, Ph.D (Editor/Contributor)** is an honors graduate (magna cum laude) of the Human Services-Criminal Justice doctoral program at Capella University. His research focus was on innovation, learning, and cooperation in police organizations and communities. After finishing his dissertation work, Dr. Engbeck completed a post-graduate program in online college teaching. A strong advocate of lifelong learning, he recently completed an MIT course in Sociological Neurobiology and is currently enrolled in a Constructionist Learning class. He is a former Deputy with the Sacramento County Probation Department and has served in both the US Marine Corps and the US Army during Desert Shield/Storm and Operation Iraqi Freedom. He has been in the security and law enforcement industry since 1979. Dr Engbeck is author of *Patrol Services for Crime-Free Communities: Methods, Procedures, Alliance, and Integration* and has several police-industry articles in press; he is a staff writer for *The Banner,* the monthly publication of the Union Kit Carson Masonic Lodge. He may be reached at jengbeck@yahoo.com.

**Terry D. Anderson, PhD.** Has served as a full-time teacher for over three decades in the areas of communication, problem management, and organizational leadership in the School of Criminology and Criminal Justice at the University of the Fraser Valley in Abbotsford, BC, Canada. He has also served as an adjunct instructor or professor at the California Command College, the Justice Institute of British Columbia, Simon Fraser University, Trinity Western University, Union Institute of Sacramento, and the University of British Columbia. Dr. Anderson has conducted executive coaching and mentoring, organization development, strategic planning, team development, and executive leadership development projects for police agencies, correctional institutions, and non-profit agencies throughout the United States and Canada. His focus is on developing strategic leadership competence that has an impact on community safety. As a speaker, Dr. Anderson has delivered practical, hard-hitting messages on leadership effectiveness for organizations such as the Canadian Association of Chiefs of Police, the California Police Chiefs Forum, the European Police Leadership Forum, and the Canadian Police College's Leadership Forum. He is author of over a dozen assessments, training, and development tools, and several books devoted to transforming leadership.

**Stacey Forges** holds a B.S. degree in Criminal Justice and a M.S. degree in Criminal Justice Administration (Chaminade University) and is a Ph.D. learner at Capella University. He is a Detective/Sergeant in the Honolulu Police Department, Narcotics/Vice Division. He has been a law enforcement officer since 1989 after being honorably discharged from the United States Navy as an Intelligence Specialist specializing in Human Intelligence (HUMINT). He served in Iraq and Afghanistan. As a law enforcement officer, he was assigned to Uniform Patrol, Specialized Services Division (SSD/SWAT) team member, Solo bike officer (motorcycle), Crime Reduction Unit (CRU), plainclothes unit, Criminal Investigation Division (CID) Major Crimes Detail, Community Affairs Division, and Narcotics Vice Division. He is currently completing his Ph.D. dissertation at Capella University, focusing his qualitative research on experiences of young adults in Hawaii who are addicted to methamphetamine.

**James E. Konopasek, Ph.D.** is a former parole/probation officer and forensic therapist. He has been a licensed polygraph examiner since 2002. He is a Professor of Criminal Justice at University of Phoenix and Missouri Southern State University, teaching criminal justice ethics. He can be reached at jkonopasek@mssu.edu.

**J. E. Ruesch**, M.S., is the founder and lead consultant of Applied Performance Group Services (APG), an independent consulting firm that specializes in enhancing individual and team performance in professional athletics, businesses, and the military. Jim retired from the U.S. Army in 2005, having served with distinction for 20 years in units such as the 12th Special Forces Group, 3rd Ranger Battalion, the U.S. Army Training and Doctrine Command, and as an instructor at the United States Military Academy at West Point. Jim is the founding director of a cutting edge program called the Army Center for Enhanced Performance where he marketed, resourced, staffed, and managed the start-up of the new program for the Department of Defense. As part of this program, Jim personally trained more than 2000 Army Special Forces soldiers at the John F. Kennedy Special Warfare Center and School. A former mixed martial artist fighter, Jim coached the Army Martial Arts Team for over seven years to national and international recognition. Today, Jim works with professional and Olympic athletes from the National Football League, Ultimate Fighting Championship, and the Olympic Training Center. He also provides services to business executives and law-enforcement agencies around the country. He can be reached at jruesch@apgsonline.com.

**Harold R. Torrens, B.A., M.A.,** is a Commander in the Cincinnati Ohio Investigative Unit, Ohio Department of Public Safety. He has been a law enforcement officer since 1990 and works with a specialized undercover unit that investigates alcohol and tobacco violations and food-stamp fraud. He has been recognized nationally as the recipient of the National Agent of the Year Award from the National Liquor Law Enforcement Association. Commander Torrens speaks professionally on the subject of gambling and synthetic narcotics investigation, and he is currently completing his Ph.D. dissertation at Capella University, focusing on prostitution and human trafficking interventions with an emphasis on demand reduction.

# Table of Contents

## Abbreviations and Acronyms

| | |
|------|------|
| AS | Anxiety Sensitivity |
| ASD | Acute Stress Disorder |
| CSF | Comprehensive Soldier Fitness |
| DSM | Diagnostic and Statistical Manual of Mental Disorders |
| EHB | Essential Healthcare Benefits |
| HRV | Heart Rate Variability |
| PERMA | Positive Emotion, Engagement, Relationships, Meaning, Achievement |
| POST | California Commission on Police Officer Standards and Training |
| PTSD | Post Traumatic Stress Disorder |
| SLT | Social Learning Theory |
| USDOJ | United States Department of Justice |
| VA | Veterans Administration |

# Foreword

*Superheroes balance the forces of light and dark, rage and serenity, and the sacred and profane within themselves and from it forge an identity that is powerful and purposeful.*

—Deepak Chopra, *The Seven Spiritual Laws of Superheroes: Harnessing Our Power to Change the World*

In his book *The Art of Possibility*, Conductor Benjamin Zander writes that there are three responses to life's circumstances: Resignation, Anger, and Possibilities. For too long the majority response to policing's well-known physical, social, and emotional challenges has been resignation or anger -- neither of which is healthy and productive. But asking "What is possible?" is liberating and hopeful. *Beyond Survival Tactics* answers "what is possible" to change the human condition of our police officers.

Since 1970 when I followed my calling to become a police officer, I have experienced and witnessed the toll that this profession takes on too many who have answered "the call." Policing is a noble calling, but the cost of spending the majority of one's adult life in service of others is well known and accepted. Yet, for my 40 plus years of serving, teaching, and consulting in policing, the comprehensive, practical, holistic solutions to our challenges seemed elusive. But they are not. The research, writing, and practices of many are now teaching us that we *can* change the condition of policing, and quite easily it seems.

The collective work of the authors of *Beyond Survival Tactics* has resulted in an indispensable book of research, resources, and best practices that can teach officers how to take command of their own well-being, performance, and life success. They have successfully blended the science with the art while mixing in extensive real-world experience.

For those in the business of leading, teaching, shaping, and molding police officers, this work will guide their path. For our men and women in blue, this work will assist as you navigate the perils of police work. Our police academies and our career in-service training have historically been exceptional in developing the requisite skills of policing. Yet we have failed to consistently develop the human capacity that is foundational to not only serving honorably but to sustaining a healthy, happy, and rewarding life while serving and in retirement.

*Beyond Survival Tactics* is about the hard work of developing the heart of the officer who wears the badge. It is body armor for the soul of a cop! Oddly, as you the reader will discover, the solutions described often do not have their roots in policing. The origins are found in new and even ancient practices: in the science of Coherence from the

Institute of HeartMath, the practices of Positive Psychology, the philosophy of excellence that leads to World Class Performance, and even the art of transforming leadership. These are just a few of the gifts the reader will gain from this journey of discovery.

Following the crash of Asiana Flight 214 in San Francisco, NTSB Chairman Deborah A. P. Hersman discussed the extensive technology and systems onboard to assist the pilot in flying and landing the plane. But she emphasized that while these systems are sophisticated and extensive "the pilot still has to fly the plane!" *Beyond Survival Tactics* is a work that informs and enlightens police officers to be the effective pilots of our own lives and careers.

The hard work of teaching us how to better care for our own health and well-being has and is continuing to be done by researchers, authors, and practitioners. We should thank them for empowering us through their work – but we still must fly the plane!

Each of us must take charge of our lives, our habits, and our health. We are responsible for serving capably and for our peak performance. We are responsible for our readiness to respond when we are tested by the crucible moments that are sure to come. That readiness begins with understanding the conditions, embracing the solutions, and -- with a focused discipline -- for developing the rituals and routines that will transform the average into the exceptional.

Enjoy the Journey and stay safe!

Commander Michael J. Nila

Commander Michael J. Nila (Ret.) developed his distinguished leadership and speaking skills while serving for 29 years in the policing profession. After retiring as a Police Commander with the Aurora, Illinois Police Department, Commander Nila joined the Blue Courage leadership development team which has provided training for such agencies the Chicago, Los Angeles, and New York City Police Departments, the U.S. Department of Justice, and the United Nations as well as the military and Fortune 500 companies. His remarkable dedication to leadership education touches hearts while it enhances self-improvement, thoughtful stress management and resilience practices, and improved overall health and well-being. Commander Nila may be reached by mail at Blue Courage, 123 South Evanslawn Avenue, Aurora, IL 60506 or through the Blue Courage website: bluecourage.com/about.html.

# Beyond Survival Tactics

## Life and Career Sustainability for Peace Officers

### Preface

This work was begun in late 2011 during the heated days of the "Occupy Movement" in the United States. Many of the potential contributors were eager to work on a book about police health and recognized the barrier-spanning potential of such an undertaking. When the editor suggested that the word "police officer" could be written as "peace keeper," ideas, questions, even contributions began drifting in with accelerating momentum. When the editor suggested that the work might also be concerned with developing compassion and empathy for fellowman, things really took form.

This work is a collaborative effort to honor the men and women who serve as peace keepers throughout the nation; and it is a work that acknowledges their dilemmas, risks, flaws and fears, and heroism. It is filled with hope for individual growth and learning within a collective and community resource pool that positively contributes to the well-being of the whole. Section 1 offers a review of research dedicated to understanding afflictions associated with high-stress occupations or lifestyles. Section 2 is a compendium of resources that may be helpful to individuals and agencies concerned with addressing and overcoming health problems. Section 3 looks at promising new directions in research and in individual endeavors to regain and maintain good health.

The work also looks at challenges and responsibilities of law enforcement agencies and their communities. It considers the notion that the law enforcement officer may be burdened with responsibilities that are best intended for the whole – the human collective known as society. If the reader will consider the issue of responsibility for a moment, while holding in abeyance any consideration of who actually "owns" this responsibility, then it may be possible to gauge the immensity of the burden. The collective and social good, even the collective's survival, seem somehow intrinsically joined in the balance of this burden. If the reader perceives the weight and/or burden of civic responsibility as emanating from everyone within society by a natural process, the weight is nothing but immense. So let's ponder who is actually tasked with upholding these responsibilities. Does the fabric of our society suggest that each member is beholden to the other, or does it offer each the individual opportunity to benefit above the other and then ask the "peace officer" to compensate? If so, what is the ratio of police people to citizens? According to the United States Bureau of Census statistics, there were nearly 900,000 sworn officers in the United States in 2008; the population of the United States is over 300 million. Is our culturally embedded institutional and societal programming set for impossibility? Not enough cops? Get more? It seems that budgets are only allowing for the opposite, and the gap is growing each day.

Is the police officer's role in the social system to simply carry some of society's burdens? Each citizen contributes to the construct of the social contract, and the role of the police practitioner may simply be to cultivate that contribution. But does he/she currently? Can he/she? The answer may be that under current conditions, the peace officer cannot effectively lead at all, but is relegated to chasing an impossible mission with after-the-fact reactions that scarcely alter the flow of events in reality. Now, let's consider the preparation police people are afforded and at the same time consider how many of us wish to live their tedium-to-trauma lifestyle; rescue a bruised, abused, and abandoned child; assist a little old lady to her cardboard home or the nearest temporary shelter; pick up the pieces and quiet the neighborhood after a ghetto gang has killed several of its members; dig among the ruins of a housing site that Mother Nature has leveled in a major earthquake . . . . If law enforcement people are willing to engage the teetering giant of collective hubris, nonchalance, and ethical negligence, they must have optimal health to have even the proverbial snowball's chance in hell. Thus, this work is intended to bolster, fortify, and "occupy" police health.

With gratitude for all who contributed so thoughtfully to this work and for individuals who supplied indispensable guidance, positive energy, and loving care,

John R. Engbeck
July 23, 2013
Garden Valley, California

# Police Health and Well-Being:

## What Do We Know About the Many Faces of Stress?

A great many researchers and theorists have offered insight into the nature of stress, among them University of Calgary Professor Emeritus Robert E. Franken (1994) who was concerned with the body's neurological and physiological adaptive functions. In stressful situations the body's sympathetic/adrenal system governs rapid-response arousal while the slower-acting pituitary/adrenal system serves to prolong activated awareness. It is clear, however, that many factors have a role in explaining the nature of stress; for example, gender differences, ethnic differences, biological vulnerability, and human perception and cognition. An event that is stressful to one individual may be a fairly routine occurrence to another. A simple example is the fire-truck siren that serves as problem-solving tool for the fireman-driver but as an emergency stress-producer for a nearby pedestrian. Moreover, stressors differ in duration, with acute stressors generally limited to short periods of time and chronic stressors activating the body's responses for prolonged periods; for example, the fire truck siren vs. grief from losing a loved one. The biopsychosocial model of stress discussed by Bernard & Krupat (1994) posited that there are three significant elements of stress: an external element that precedes and triggers a stress response; an internal element involving individual neurological, physiological, and psychological reactions; and a recognizable interaction between the two.

For the most part, this work treats stress as a situational imbalance in which events or perceived demands place strains on individuals, communities, and societies. Not all stress reactions are negative, of course, as they activate arousal, mobilize efforts, and maximize the expenditure of energy to prepare the body to meet challenging situations. They are, in fact, necessary for survival. The risk of disease is heightened when extreme stress impacts the body's hormone-control centers and creates chemical imbalances that impact

3

the nervous and endocrine systems. Cortisol, a biomarker of stress, is the major hormone the body secretes during stressful situations. Its normal pattern is to become elevated as a person wakes from sleep, to level off throughout the day, and to decrease at night. Under conditions of extreme stress, however, the pattern may be seriously disrupted; the response becomes maladaptive when the body's reaction is not healthfully controlled by normal regulatory mechanisms. (Please see Appendix, page 113, for a definition of terms used in this work.)

## Looking at Medusa

In Greek mythology, Medusa was a hideous-looking monster with human female attributes but with masses of poisonous, living snakes in place of hair. To look directly at her would turn a person to stone. By viewing Medusa in his polished shield, the hero Perseus was able to slay her, and he eventually gave the head of Medusa to Athena to place on her shield. Medusa was, thus, both a life-threatening entity and a guardian-protectress — a symbol of life energy. A barrage of distractions, disruptions, interruptions, challenges, family worries, financial worries, work-place pressures, unmet deadlines, physical threats, emergencies . . . that contribute to stress overload in our lives may in fact be eroding our ability to learn and to remember. Below is a compilation of self-reported symptoms attributed to stress by peace officers.

> **Fatigue/Muscle tremors/Vomiting/Grinding of teeth/ Nausea/Profuse sweating/Chest pain/Rapid heart rate/Twitches/Difficulty breathing/ Dizziness/ Diarrhea/Blackouts/Headaches/Panic attacks/ Depression/Insomnia/ Emotional outbursts/Substance abuse/Impaired memory**

Elevated stress reactions in peace officers assuredly create personal, community, medical, political, and financial burdens. Using the gift of academic research as a polished shield, let's take a look at the monster stress to see its many manifestations and then to see how we may regenerate life energy from knowledge and mindful attention to our health issues.

While the body's stress responses enable people to react quickly to threatening situations, it is clear that heavy stress load impairs health. But until recently specific mechanisms of stress-related disease and dysfunction were foggy or undetermined. Research by Koo and Duman (2008) determined the key receptor in the brain that is critical in the harm cycle. The research supports a fairly well known concept in pharmacology, psychiatry, and neuroscience, which is that uncontrollable stress can be linked to changes in the cellular structure of the brain itself and the hippocampus in particular, which appears to be uniquely vulnerable to stress factors. The researchers found that stress hormones and related biochemical effects worked in unison to actually deter the hippocampus from building new cells. The specific receptor, called the IL-1B cytokine receptor, may cause a mitigation of the sensation of pleasure, and stress that is relative to the receptor also harmfully affects the brain in the hypothalamus, the adrenal system, and the pituitary gland. The researchers also explored means to influence the receptors' functions and diminish the brain-cell destructive cycle. The Veterans Administration and the National Center for Post Traumatic Stress Disorder were among the agencies funding the research.

Research relating specifically to stress among peace officers (Gershon, et al., 2000) intended to measure perceived work stress among police officers in correlation with officer health and stress coping-mechanisms. Over 1,000 officers in an urban force responded to a survey questionnaire relating to such issues as workplace environments, discrimination and lack of cooperation, levels of job satisfaction, exposure to emergencies, officer-safety issues, personal and professional relationships, and more. The study found that organizational stressors, not critical incidents, were most strongly associated with perceived stress. The researchers found a strong association between perceived stress and negative behavior such as spousal abuse, aggression, and increased alcohol use. The study also noted that officers who reported high levels of stress were at increased risk of health problems and suggested that coping styles that focus on positive actions — as opposed to avoidance and/or self-condemnation and shame, for example — were most effective in reducing adverse health outcomes. In addition, the study found that interventions that modify certain *accessible* stressors can bolster resilience and support effective coping and effective police-health reform.

Critical-incident scenario enactments were used in a recent study by Groer, et al (2010) to gauge biopsychological reactions and effects on health. The biomarkers that were used were based on salivary levels of over 100 police participants, and scenario incidents were designed to evoke high levels of stress. They were implemented with the intend of analyzing difference responses to disparate situations. One scenario enactment, for example, was brief and involved the police person's own mortality, while another was extended over a longer time span and involved a serious, but non-lethal, threat to lives. The saliva tests examined secretions of immunoglobulin as well as cortisol and some additional concentrations of biological composition such as interleukin- 6 and alpha amylase formations. The extended scenario resulted in higher reactions than the brief life-taking scenario, suggesting that duration of stress exposure is a significant factor as is incident-related stress that endangers not only self, but others as well. The research affords perspectives on connections between the conscious mind and the body wherein an enacted scenario results in hard physiological ramifications. Such scenario enactment may be useful in developing self-awareness and stress-reduction skills.

## Gender Variation in Stress Responses

Research conducted during the first decade of the twenty-first century was unusually rich for individuals and agencies attempting to understand the complexities of human interactions and to consider how they might constructively transform situations relating to police health and well-being. Among the treasures of this period was an important research project conducted at University of Pennsylvania School of Medicine that found fundamental differences among men and women's stress responses, as different parts of the brain activate during performance-related stress testing. Neurology Professor J.J. Wang (2007) led the research project, and readers with sufficient understanding of human physiology may enjoy reading the full research report as well as a National Institute of Mental Health report on how chronic stress may be linked to such ailments as anxiety disorders, depression, and PTSD (Du, et al., 2009), which revealed how individual cells adapt to deal with sudden or extreme challenges and how chronic stress may reduce cell plasticity and resilience.

Focusing specifically on stress among police officers, a pilot study of the Buffalo Cardio-metabolic Occupational Police Stress (Violanti, et al., 2006) integrated psychological, physiological, and subclinical measures of stress, disease, and mental dysfunction among 100 officers in the Buffalo, New York police department One perhaps startling result of the study was the finding that 16 percent of the officers met criteria for depression, and 36 percent reported elevated PTSD symptoms. While this 2006 study was not specifically concerned with gender differences, Dr. Violanti (2009) and team later examined chronic stress among members of a mid-sized urban law enforcement department, focusing specifically on the associations between cortisol and brachial artery reactions as they relate to cardiovascular disease. The random sample of officers was stratified on gender, with 33 percent of the participants being female. Elevated cortisol secretion after awakening was significantly associated with impaired artery flow mediated dilation in women, while a similar result was not found among male officers. This research adds to our understanding of gender difference in stress response, and, again, readers with understanding of human physiology may wish to examine the research methods and detailed findings at this website: www. ncbi.nlm.nih.gov/pubmed/19616310.

Related research work by University of California Psychology Professor Shelley E. Taylor et al. (2000 and 2008) examined biobehavioral responses to stress among women and the neural bases of cortisol stress responses. In the earlier work, Taylor and team coined the phrase "tend-and-befriend" to describe stress responses experienced by women, pointing out that earlier research on "flight-or-fight" responses was concerned primarily with human male responses.

7

The researchers concluded that females under stress tend to nurture and protect themselves and their young and to form alliances with others. They suggested that hormones may be significant in explaining male and female dimensions of stress responses; males experiencing stress produce androgens such as testosterone and stress hormones such as cortisol, while females under stress produce oxytocin which may reduce fear and decrease some elements of the flight-or-flight response. According to Azar (2000), the tend-and-befriend response builds on the brain's attachment/caregiving system, which may counteract the metabolic activity of the fight-or-flight response.

Additional research by McCarty, Zhao, & Garland (2007) examined burnout and occupational stress in men and women police officers, suggesting that men and women engaged in police work may have differing levels of resiliency. Some of the independent variables used in the study included coping mechanisms in normal use, other demographically influenced variables, and ranges of common coping mechanisms. The research revealed that there are differences amidst the variance of gender, particularly as regards Black American females who reported significantly higher levels of burnout. The researchers pointed out that the study was limited in focus to a single police department. Nevertheless, the results support a generalizable view that special consideration of police officers as individuals may be fruitful.

More recently, researchers at Harvard University School of Public Health (Kloog, et al., 2011) found a link between sleeping habits and risks of developing hormonal cancer. The study involved 1679 women and their exposure to light at night and in their sleeping habitat. The research revealed that shiftwork that involves sleep deprivation and disruption of circadian rhythm is a risk factor for breast cancer.

*The "Hardiness" Factor.* Readers may enjoy a research report by Michael E. Andrew, et al. (2008) who were interested in individual responses to stress among 105 randomly selected police officers (40 women and 65 men). The researchers looked at hardiness factors — commitment, control and challenge — in association with depression, PTSD, and general psychological distress. Analyses were stratified by gender, and the study found that, with regard to depression and PTSD symptoms, the *commitment* dimension of hardiness may be more protective in female officers than in male officers. Hardiness *commitment* was negatively associated with the psychological distress scale for both men and women The hardiness *control* dimension was significantly and negatively associated with depression for both genders but was not associated with PTSD.

The American Psychological Association (2011) has produced several news releases that highlight gender-related attitudes about stress management. The following chart summarizes some of those observations.

---

**Observations on Stress Management**

-Men appear more reluctant than women to recognize relationships between stress and health.

-Men place less emphasis on stress management than women do.

-Women report higher levels of stress than men do.

-Women are more likely than men to consider lifestyle or behavior changes to manage stress.

-Men are more likely than women to report diagnosis of high blood pressure, type 2 diabetes, and heart disease or heart attack.

-One in four women acknowledge they are not doing enough to manage stress; only 17 percent of men feel this way.

-Both men (65 percent) and women (66 percent) say they are generally satisfied with their lives, but only 45 percent of men and 44 percent of women report satisfaction with their financial security.

-Men are less likely than women to say they are doing an excellent or very good job handling relationships with family and friends, eating healthfully, and getting enough sleep.

-Men are more likely to rely on playing sports for stress management while women report using a multitude of strategies such as reading, spending time with family, praying, going to religious services, shopping, getting a massage, or seeing a mental -health professional.

---

Several studies summarized in the following pages distinguish between male and female participants and characteristics. Of particular interest may be a research report on decision-making styles among police investigators (Salo & Allwood, 2011) discussed on page 24. Also see Violanti et al. (2007) on obesity and depression, page 20, and Violanti, (2010) on suicide, page 21.

## Post Traumatic Stress Disorder and Police Health

It may be useful to begin a discussion of post traumatic stress disorder (PTSD) with a look at the American Psychiatric Association publication *Diagnostic and Statistical Manual of Mental Disorders* (DSM), which is intended to provide researchers, clinicians, pharmaceutical and insurance companies, and policy and regulation agencies with common language and criteria for classifying mental disorders. The diagnostic tool is reproduced on the following page.

The advent of PTSD is commonly a reaction to having experienced a life-threatening event and/or witnessed a traumatic and life-threatening event, according to Psychiatrist Ben Green (2009), whose research used psychiatric measures to analyze PTSD symptoms and effects. Police officers who acquire the disorder may often exhibit symptoms of depression, anxiety, avoidance, flashbacks, and hyper-arousal states. A key component of PTSD is its potential to harm the officer's ability to concentrate and/or to pay direct and extended attention. Other aspects of the affliction affect the functioning of the brain's central lobe, and victims of PTSD may be limited in their ability to think in abstractions, which can cause all manner of issues when rapid-response judgments are required. Physiological symptoms also may include hypertension and nervous-system issues while also creating a blockage to the officer's insight into a particular dilemma.

The complications include incidences where many victims of PTSD may not see the need for treatment and/or deny the condition and thus confound the treatment scenario inexorably. It is quite possible that a diagnosis of PTSD might compel the department to re-orchestrate the employment arrangement; thus, law enforcement personnel may be the last to accept treatment but among the most needful. Green recommends that sufferers seek full and complete treatment.

# Diagnostic Criteria for PTSD

**A. The person has been exposed to a traumatic event in which both of the following were present:**

1. the person experienced, witnessed, or was confronted with an event or events that involved actual or threatened death or serious injury, or a threat to the physical integrity of self or others.

2. the person's response involved intense fear, helplessness, or horror. **Note**: In children, this may be expressed instead by disorganized or agitated behavior.

**B. The traumatic event is persistently reexperienced in one (or more) of the following ways:**

1. recurrent and intrusive distressing recollections of the event, including images, thoughts, or perceptions. **Note**: In young children, repetitive play may occur in which themes or aspects of the trauma are expressed.

2. recurrent distressing dreams of the event. **Note**: In children, there may be frightening dreams without recognizable content.

3. acting or feeling as if the traumatic event were recurring (includes a sense of reliving the experience, illusions, hallucinations, and dissociative flashback episodes, including those that occur on awakening or when intoxicated). Note: In young children, trauma-specific reenactment may occur.

4. intense psychological distress at exposure to internal or external cues that symbolize or resemble an aspect of the traumatic event.

5. physiological reactivity on exposure to internal or external cues that symbolize or resemble an aspect of the traumatic event.

**C. Persistent avoidance of stimuli associated with the trauma and numbing of general responsiveness (not present before the trauma), as indicated by three (or more) of the following:**

1. efforts to avoid thoughts, feelings, or conversations associated with the trauma.

2. efforts to avoid activities, places, or people that arouse recollections of the trauma.

3. inability to recall an important aspect of the trauma.

4. markedly diminished interest or participation in significant activities.

5. feeling of detachment or estrangement from others.

6. restricted range of affect (e.g., unable to have loving feelings).

7. sense of a foreshortened future (e.g., does not expect to have a career, marriage, children, or a normal life span).

**D. Persistent symptoms of increased arousal (not present before the trauma), as indicated by two (or more) of the following:**

1. difficulty falling or staying asleep.

2. irritability or outbursts of anger.

3. difficulty concentrating.

4. Hypervigilance.

5. exaggerated startle response.

**E. Duration of the disturbance (symptoms in Criteria B, C, and D) is more than 1 month.**

**F. The disturbance causes clinically significant distress or impairment in social, occupational, or other important areas of functioning.**

**Specify if: Acute:** if duration of symptoms is less than 3 months. **Chronic**: if duration of symptoms is 3 months or more

**Specify if:** With Delayed Onset: if onset of symptoms is at least 6 months after the stressor.

Source: DSM-IV-TR:

www1.appstate.edu/~hillrw/PTSD%20CBT%20TX/PTSD/Pages/Diagnositics.htm.)

Site created by Jenn Andrus.

***Why Me?*** Many researchers have sought information about identifiable precursors to PTSD and about beneficial preemptive health measures. Research by Yuan et al. (2011) was conducted to develop information about how and why some police officers exposed to traumatic incidents develop chronic conditions and symptoms of PTSD while other officers do not. The research sought out potentially protective factors that might be part of the reason for the disparities among police sample populations. The incidence of PTSD development in a sample of over 200 police officers showed that factors such as benevolent beliefs, social support and adjustment, race, and also smaller degrees of exposure to traumatic and/or critical incidents were all apparent correlates of lower PTSD likelihood. The research used the NEO Five-Factor Personality Inventory and was conducted longitudinally beginning with basic academy surveys and ending with a two-year span of service behind the same officers. The work garnered the strong inferential conclusion that positive and benevolent belief systems and social-adjustment skills, strong social support systems, and a strong sense of self-worth were predictive of lower-risk PTSD development. The findings support continuing efforts to understand PTSD and to pre-mitigate its persistence among police officers; findings also suggest that consciousness and awareness play pivotal roles in the preventing development of PTSD.

Prior to the Yuan study, researchers with the New York Academy of Sciences examined traits and characteristics in peace officers that might be indicative of later PTSD onset (Marmar et al., 2006). Resilience and risk factors associated with PTSD in the study were extensive and included level of vulnerability to peritraumatic panic attacks; various preclinical studies on extinction and fear conditioning were considered as well. The research indicated that there are recognizable individual differences in PTSD resilience The traits that appeared to be predictive for PTSD in terms of resilience or vulnerability included skills with problem-solving and coping, level of peritraumatic distress, amount of peritraumatic dissociation, level of work-environment stress, and level of social support.

***Measuring Dimensions of PTSD.*** Understanding of PTSD was further enhanced by research conducted by academic researchers G. J. Asmundson and J. A. Stapleton (2008) who examined symptom severity and associations between anxiety sensitivity(AS), such as psychological, social, and somatic concerns, and empirically supported PTSD symptoms, such as re-experiencing, avoidance, numbing, and hyperarousal. The study involved a sample of 138 police officers who had all reported experiencing an event they perceived as traumatic. Forty-four screened positive for PTSD. Participants with probable PTSD scored significantly higher on AS total concerns, and AS somatic concerns were significant predictors of PTSD total symptom severity. Only depressive symptoms were significant predictors of numbing and hyperarousal cluster scores. The study included implications for treatment of individuals with and without panic-related symptoms.

Research work conducted by Professors Brian Chopko (a mental health counselor and former police officer) and Robert C. Schwartz (2009) focused on the reactions of first responders who experienced high levels of trauma-related stress, which often is associated with emotional and social sufferings that include anxiety, substance abuse, thoughts of suicide, job "burn-out", memory impairment, and PTSD. Other related physical problems included cardiovascular, neurological, gastrointestinal, audiological, and pain symptoms. Consistent with other findings, the researchers found that spiritual growth was a factor in lower risk post-traumatic growth. Further study conducted by Professor Chopko (2010) and using the Impact of Events Scale-Revised indicated that situations involving officers in duty-related shootings became a predictor of post-traumatic growth.

Research by Anke B. Witteveen et al. (2006) examined stress responses among fire and police personnel who had been involved in an air disaster event. The research was intended to evaluate two self-report scales: The Impact of Event Scale (IES) using four factors (intrusion, avoidance, emotional numbing, and sleep disturbance) and the Self-Rating Inventory for Post-traumatic Stress Disorder (SRIP), using five factors (intrusion, avoidance, hyperarousal, emotional numbing and sleep disturbance). The research discovered correlations between the reactions of both high- and low-level-affected subjects, particularly in terms of numbing and avoidance responses. The validity and reliability of the measurements and their process of inquiry were shown to be high and resolute, while the relationship between similar factors in both instruments was only low to moderate.

Witteveen et al. (2010) later studied nearly 2000 police officers and firefighters to examine the correlation between cortisol levels and PTSD. Researchers had correlated cortisol and PTSD among various groups of subjects, but inconsistent associations created barriers to defining a clear linear relationship. In the Witteveen study, researchers incorporated such variables as negatively affective life events and exposure to disaster, as well as salivary-control levels in correlation with stress and PTSD. Negative-event exposure was shown to have a high correlation with PTSD and cortisol levels as well as sleep disturbance outcomes. The researchers attempted to mitigate the confounding variables associated with the measurements to arrive at a best-possible statistical-confidence level. In a final estimation, a basis of 10% influence was determined between PTSD and the glandular activities, a finding that establishes a causal path.

## Sleep, Performance, and Well-Being

*Sleep that knits up the ravell'd sleeve of care, . . sore labour's bath, balm of hurt minds, great nature's second course, chief nourisher in life's feast.*
William Shakespeare, *Macbeth*, *Act II, scene 2.*

Various studies have established that workers in police, fire, military, aviation and medical-based occupations encounter stressors that may have negative impact on quality of sleep; likewise, sleep disturbance negatively impacts performance and health. Moreover, sleep deprivation symptoms are varied, and many sufferers remain undiagnosed and/or untreated. Considering the potentially severe consequences of fatigue-related errors, Dr. Tom Neylan et al. (2002) studied over 700 large-city police officers in relation to critical-incident stressors as well as routine stress exposure. Compared to civilian control groups, police officers reported greater incidence of sleep disturbance, diminished sleep quality, and less sleep time. Nightmares were associated with critical-incident exposure, but there was only a weak association with insomnia. By contrast, general work-related stresses were associated with insomnia. In a later study, Dr. Neylan et al. (2010) examined the relationships between sleep and fatigue-related errors in psychomotor performance. The study focused specifically on whether or not relationships between prior-night-sleep duration and performance of psychomotor tasks could be detected. Healthy police-academy recruits were the subjects of the seven-day field study of sleep-wake activity and changes in reaction time. The psychomotor vigilance factors for the recruits were assessed against differing levels of responses during the 1,000 nights of sleep being studied. Logistical regression techniques were used to expose the possible influence of the prior night's sleep-health factor. Propensity for error dropped with sound sleep the night before the test; moreover, error propensity decreased over time since the subjects' waking regardless of prior night's sleep. The study corroborated linkage between cognitive performance and circadian rhythm and established that relationships between prior-night-sleep duration and performance of psychomotor tasks could be detected.

A recorded interview with Dr. Neylan (2007) revealed that researchers have uncovered many correlations between sleep and health, particularly where sleep provides a restorative process to the bio-psycho-physiological organism. The relationships between sleep, good sleep, and sleep deprivation has been examined many times over, but Dr. Neylan's work suggests that insomnia could be a leading, if not *the* leading, health challenge to police work and to healthful, sustainable human existence in general. Neylan's research work at the San Francisco Veterans Affairs Medical Center has added insights into the kinds of health risks poor sleep actually may cause and/or exacerbate. Neylan asserted that the PTSD and hypervigilance symptoms of many veterans are related to their disrupted sleep patterns. He also held that sleep and restorative cycles within the body are parts of the animal world without exception, as they are perhaps parts of a universal cycle of night and day. Human circadian rhythms are innate within our biological structure, and the human brain is a highly susceptible target for the ravages of sleep deprivation. The effects of poor sleep are well documented in relation to many types of diseases and maladies and are particularly significant in relation to heart disease, aging, and blood pressure. In addition, the disabling effects of sleep deprivation have been tied to weight-control failures and metabolic shifts, suggesting that important balances are upset by sleep shortage.

The balances of human energy flows are also a key to understanding complex relationships tied to chronic insomnia and stress. The incidence of anxiety is key, and it opens inquiry into a particularly likely path. The hormonal secretions that occur as part of anxiety provide a means of developing and enhancing our understanding of sleep and general health. Our primordial capability to fend off sleep for immediate survival necessities may lurk in our modern paradigm without good cause and to our detriment for the most part if we are hyper vigilant of imagined threats in the "jungle". Neylan also mentioned the incidence of corticotropin release and how it has been shown to depreciate healthful sleep patterns. The call is to examine this paradigm of sleep and health much more vigorously and to examine a contention that all health concerns may relate to the restorative factors of good sleep. Humans apparently crave and flourish from contact with other humans, and sleep shortages tend to cause isolation and avoidance, which only further the conundrum and confound the issue. Indeed, Neylan's works demonstrate connections between human intelligence level/social satisfaction/and PTSD resilience.

Dr. Bryan Vila (2006), senior researcher at Washington State University's Sleep and Performance Research Center, studied the impact of shift work or long and irregular work hours on police officers and their communities. Conditions such as fluctuating sleep patterns, emergency situations, and the influx of unstable psycho-physiological conditions associated with police work appear to be fertile soil for mental health threats, psychological dysfunction, and dysfunctional relationship woes. The research focused on both mental and physical fatigue, with emphasis on the former and with information regarding the potential costs of treatment and the associated costs related to performance, decision-making, and safety issues. The Vila study asserted a causal connection between occupational performance and shift work or long, uneven hours for police people and suggested that mitigating deleterious conditions is a possible by way of enhancing programmatic police-health awareness and reform. Ever-increasing budget shortfalls, issues with recruiting and retention, and ever-escalating management demands all contribute to a potentially worsening situation. The sometimes hidden, but extreme, costs of negligence suggest that preemptive and proactive measures are overdue.

It is not surprising that patrol officers who are suffering fatigue may contribute negatively to human encounters because of impaired capability and decreased alertness. Moreover, the circadian disruptions, lack of adequate sleep and rest, and mood dysfunctions associated with lack of sleep have been linked to misconduct in some studies. In addition, fatigue generally disrupts healthy relationships with community stakeholders, family members, and fellow officers. To evaluate the effects of fatigue on police patrol officers, the Police Executive Research Forum (PERF) funded research conducted by Vila, et al. (2000) who found that many law enforcement agencies do not limit hours of work. Officers seek/accept overtime work to increase their income, and some departments support this activity because it may enhance long-term retention opportunities and alleviate some staffing issues. Nevertheless, the deployment of fatigued officers in law enforcement may be as much as six times higher than in other regulated industries where safety is an acknowledged concern. With regard to over-time hours spent in court appearances, the judiciary body of the government does not directly pay the added costs and may have little cause to acknowledge fatigue issues.

The PERF report showed that misuse of force, officer stress, non-optimal decision making, and fatigue undermine the potential for community-policing success and the fragile condition of police-citizen interactions. Problem solving, particularly in public relations situations, is harmed by fatigue and sleeplessness as is individual initiative, according to Vila et al. High adrenalin situations may be thought to alleviate fatigue, but research shows that fatigue actually accelerates after the adrenal push subsides. An additional concern of the report was the fact that partners of fatigued officers may be in jeopardy. Heightened fearfulness and irritability are elements of debilitating fatigue situations.

The Vila team used a pupilometer to examine fatigue in officers and found that 6.2 percent of the officers were clinically impaired, *as if they had consumed alcohol and were exhibiting a blood alcohol level of .10.* The team also applied the Pittsburgh Sleep Quality Index and found that 41 percent of examined officers exhibited sleep dysfunction pathologies. Clearly, poor health-care undermines the ability of patrol people to perform and reduces their educational drive and thus the ability of departments to grow and learn.

The research team of Professors Scott Senjo and Karla Dhungana (2009) made similar observations after surveying law enforcement agency directors about policies that relate to fatigue and job performance. They found a low-level desire among directors to instigate fatigue-reduction policies. In some situations, informal controls were in place. Where fatigue-reduction policies existed, researchers found emphasis on managerial conceptualization rather than on safety or civil liability orientations.

*Injury Incidence.* Because of insufficient sleep, fatigue, erratic shift hours, and high-activity level, police officers working a midnight shift may be more injury prone than officers on either day or afternoon shifts. Using computerized payroll records from a mid-sized urban police agency and covering the years 1994 to 2010, medical researchers (Violanti et al., 2012) studied injury incidence among 430 officers. Their startling findings indicate that the incidence rate ratio of the midnight shift was 72 percent greater than the day shift, and 66 percent greater than the afternoon shift. Moreover, incidence of injury on the first night back at work was 69 percent larger than the day shift. The researchers used an age-adjusted incidence rate ratio for injury and concluded that night shift work among police officers was indeed associated with higher injury risk.

*Sleep* and *PTSD: Deciphering Causality.* Sleep provides a vital restorative and healing opportunity for humans throughout a vast range of maladies; however, with regard to PTSD, it may not yet be clear whether PTSD causes sleep dysfunction, whether sleep dysfunction causes/exacerbates PTSD, and/or whether the two disorders interact to propel each other into a disruptive and destructive cycle (Spoormaker & Montgomery, 2008). Some widely held notions suggest that PTSD causes sleep disturbances that can be mitigated by treatment of PTSD. But recent studies by Spoormaker and Montgomery have suggested that sleep disturbances have a direct potentially linear effect upon PTSD. Their research also indicated that successful treatment of PTSD has not alleviated all symptoms of sleep dysfunction in many cases, inferring that the causal connection is not solely or directionally linear. Sleep research has confirmed positive effects of sleep on PTSD conditions, which further supports the proposition that the relationship is at least a two-way street. Rapid-eye-movement (REM) studies may reveal more about the association of PTSD and sleep dysfunction. A key takeaway from these observations is that healthful sleep is instrumental in PTSD treatment and that PTSD contributes conversely. Preemptive sleep-function measurements may assist in treatment of both PTSD and sleep dysfunction.

## Connecting the Dots: Depression . . . Metabolic Syndrome . . . Cardio-Vascular Issues . . . Obesity . . . Suicide

Police work rates as one of the most stressful occupations in society, and it is fraught with health issues. The constancy of trauma and stress conditions in police work make it fertile soil for the specter of depression and its symptomatic implications to take hold. University researchers at the Shanghai Mental Health Center in China (Wang, et al., 2010) examined stress predictors over time, utilizing a sample population of approximately 120 police-officer recruits. The research combined measures ranging from childhood traumatic-event exposure to neuroticism and the self-worth scale for pre-event inquiry as well as post-event longitudinal measures of negative life-events, critical-incident exposure, conditions of PTSD and anxiety, and more. The testing differentiated between depressive symptoms and PTSD symptoms to provide insight into precursor behaviors and possible early treatment. The correlations that were found suggested linearly opposing relationships between a rising self-worth and previous trauma, and the findings strongly suggested that reduction in work-place stress for police officers can reduce duty-related depression. Questions that arise from these findings are: If police people who serve across the nation are valued by the society they serve and protect, what is society doing about the potential for depression in its servants, and what holds the industry back from understanding and remedies?

*Metabolic syndrome* is an aggregation of risk factors that heighten the risk for coronary artery disease, stroke, and type-2 diabetes. All of the risks are related to obesity, and the risk factors have also been associated with psychological conditions. Individuals suffering from metabolic syndrome typically have extra weight around their waists (a useful preliminary screening tool), and they may also experience excess blood clotting and low levels of inflammation throughout the body. According to Professor Scott Grundy (2008), individuals with metabolic syndrome have twice the risk for cardiovascular disease compared with those without the syndrome and five times the risk for type-2 diabetes. His study of worldwide incidence of metabolic syndrome focused on obesity and sedentary life habits as the root of the problem.

In an earlier study of police trauma and cardiovascular disease, Dr. John Violanti, et al. (2006) sought to establish associations between PTSD symptoms and metabolic syndrome among officers. The researchers considered the metabolic syndrome to be present if three or more of these symptoms were exhibited: obesity, high blood pressure, reduced high-density lipoprotein cholesterol, elevated triglycerides, and abnormal glucose levels. The study considered subclinical, mild, moderate, and severe PTSD symptom levels and found that metabolic syndrome was three times more likely to affect officers with severe PTSD symptoms. In a related study of atypical work hours and metabolic syndrome among police officers, Violanti et al. (2009) found that shorter sleep duration and more overtime along with mid-night shift work may contribute to the metabolic syndrome.

*Cardiovascular Disease and Police Stress.* University researchers Warren Franke et al. (2010) sought to determine the connections between cardiopulmonary and cardiovascular disease and stress in police work. The job-related stresses of police work were analyzed in correlation with biophysiological indicators such as mediating vascular anti-inflammatories. The sampling and data collection included responses regarding exhaustion, police perceptions of stress, strain from on-the-job stressors, perception of inequity and/or organizational chaos, and perceived supports from the agency culture. Six hundred police personnel were polled with roughly 65 percent of those being sworn personnel. The findings depicted a causal correlation between heart disease and police work but could not convincingly identify the specific and/or direct causal agent to be chronic work-related stress above other potentially inflammatory components. During the previous year, a research team (Joseph et al. 2009) reported on a study of police work and subclinical atherosclerosis, finding that urban peace officers, compared to the population sample, had elevated levels of cardiovascular disease risk factors (blood pressure, cholesterol levels, and smoking prevalence).

*Obesity and Depression.* Possible association between measures of obesity and depression was examined by Violanti et al. (2007) in a cross-sectional observational study of 115 police officers stratified by gender and randomly selected from an urban police department. Measures of obesity were body mass index, abdominal height, and waist circumference. The Center for Epidemiological Studies Depression (CES-D) Scale was used to screen for depressive symptoms and behaviors. (The self-reporting screening scale was developed by L. S. Radloff and is available at the website www.counsellingresource.com/lib/quizzes/depression-testing/cesd/). The study found a positive association in men (61 participants) between the depressive symptoms scale and both the body mass index and abdominal height, while no significant associations were found between the CES-D scale and obesity in women (42 participants). Covariate adjustments were made for age, alcohol use, years of police service, smoking, physical activity, fasting, serum glucose, and marital status, and adjustments for the covariates did not produce meaningful changes in the results. The researchers suggested additional research into other physiological and psychological factors that might influence association results.

*New Measures of Stress Responses in Police Officers.*
Research by Seattle University Professor Matthew J. Hickman and team (Hickman, et al., 2011) was conducted to seek to overcome limitations from previous studies using self-report survey data. The researchers applied new models and measurements including methods that gathered heart rate during work shifts. The factor of stress has been shown to correlate with heart rate and therefore the study's premise is well founded in other research, particularly from medical research methodologies. The context of space-time was used to gauge individual-officer heart rate and stress levels and coincidence. The research provided insight into the when, where, why of police-officer stress conditions gauging from real and unconscious reactions during actual shift events. Various implications and inferences arose from this research not the least of which may be that the methods prevalently in police research may be morphing onto more scientifically integrated and resolute terms. Moreover, Hickman et al (2011) discovered a correlation between sleep and stress in police officer performance during actual shift work to be represented by heart rate fluctuations that must be followed up with similar inquiries.

*Stress, Depression, and Genetics.* Dr. David Mrazek, professor of psychiatry and chairman of the Department of Psychiatry and Psychology at Mayo Clinic recently (Mrazek, 2011) offered historical perspective on research concerned with the relationships among stress, genetics, and depression. Dr. Mrazek related a number of studies examining depressive illness and addressing the question of why one individual manages to cope with stressful situations while another may develop mood disorders. There were research indications that individuals with a genetic variant of the serotonin transporter gene were more apt to experience depression after experiencing stressful situations. There then followed a period of debate and disagreement about these findings until a thorough analysis of 56 research studies concluded that individuals with the "less active form of the serotonin transporter gene were more vulnerable to developing depression when they experienced severe stress." The important analysis established that there is a biological vulnerability to depression and that stress may trigger its onset.

*Suicide.* National police suicide rates were compared with rates among firefighters and military personnel by Dr. John Violanti (2010). Additionally, the work examined suicide by women and minority officers. The study used the National Occupational Mortality Surveillance data between 1984 and 1998 and calculated proportionate mortality ratios. The study found that police suicide rate was four times that of firefighters. Minority officers had four and one half times the number of suicides than firefighters did, and female officers showed 12 times the number of firefighter suicides. The study also revealed that police officer suicides outnumbered homicides by 2.36 times. Dr. Violanti cautioned that the data in the study was descriptive only and that the findings do not reveal a causal relationship between police work and suicide. Nevertheless, he concluded that prevention efforts, suicide-awareness training, and psychological assistance to officers were advisable. He also recommended further research into root causes of police-officer suicides.

Covering a later time period and working with Badge of Life member Andrew F. O'Hara, Dr. Violanti (O'Hara & Violanti, 2009) sought to gather verifiable data on police suicides in order to enhance good health in the law enforcement community and to support the meaningful development of programs that address problems of police stress and suicide. They conducted the National Surveillance of Police Suicide Study in 50 states during the period January 1 to December 31, 2008, finding that there were 141 police suicides during the period, with the highest incidence in ages 35-39. Additionally, they found that service time with highest incidence was 10-14 years. Sixty-four percent of the suicides were considered "a surprise". In order to verify methodology, the researchers repeated the study in the year 2009, finding similar results with an increase in number of police suicides to 143 during the year. Other slight differences were a shift in highest risk group from ages 35-39 to ages 40-44. Twenty-seven percent of all suicides were in this age group. Similarly, there was a shift upward in service-time results, from 10-14 years of service to 20 years and above.

*Badge of Life* is an organization of active and retired police officers, medical professionals, and surviving families of suicides who are dedicated to supporting police-officer mental health, promoting healthier police forces, encouraging improved quality of service, and improving officer safety. The foundation of the organization is a suicide prevention program called the "Emotional Selfcare Program." Compete information about the program is available at www.badgeoflife.com/aboutus.php.

*Blue Courage* is another organization of police officers who are dedicated to leadership development and support for evolved police officers who are prepared at any moment to reflect the best of what policing demands. Information about the program is available at the website: http://bluecourage.com/about.html or by mail:

> **Blue Courage**
> **123 South Evanslawn Avenue**
> **Aurora, IL 60506**

The direction of change in many police agencies has been away from a reactive, hierarchical structures toward community policing visions, structures, and practices. Psychology professor J. Kevin Ford (2007) conducted a case study of a police agency moving toward a community-policing model with the intent of improving delivery of police services and becoming a learning organization. The study focused on leadership efforts to build capacity for sustaining change during the various phases of the transformation: incorporating systems thinking, eliminating command-and-control mindsets, and developing skills to support learning and improvement. The research asserted that continuous learning and change must be supported by preemptively creating supports and ongoing measures and by instituting an organizational culture that is accustomed to change and that engages change productively.

One of the challenges to these objectives lies in situations wherein institutional goals appear at odds; for example, many modern police agencies have counter terror, community policing, and emergency preparedness considerations that may contend with one another (Ford, Weissbein, & Plammondon, 2003). There are also variables in agencies, in their target learners, in politics, and, of course, in economics, that challenge organizations' ability to change. Ford et al. created a useful engagement process that depicted flow stages of organizational change: Information and reassurance, monitoring and accountability, strategic formulation, cooperation and teamwork, and co-production and empowerment. It is clear that in order to reach the high end of the chart, individuals and agencies need to be thinking clearly and solving problems critically in order to take on change.

Three of the dimensional keys to successful change, according to Ford et al. are evaluative factors such as efficiency, effectiveness, and equity. The framework exists to support officers and organizations through major changes at the institutional and organizational levels, but also on the personal level where all that change actually occurs prior to amalgam and perhaps simply in the form of resilience. Curiously, one definition of resilience is to reform after deformation, which sounds a bit like an habituated reaction, but mindful police agencies can form and reform by avoiding the unplayable situations that resistance to change creates. It is interesting that police agencies do not necessarily have a policy mandate to change, but many recognize that there is a survival mandate.

*Anticipating Workplace Change.* Work by university researchers Jana Greubel and Goran Kecklund (2010) sought information on how several kinds of organizational change impacted elements of police psychological, emotional, and bio-psychophysiological health, specifically work-related stress, sleep, recovery,and general health. The researchers also looked at how anticipation of change might affect police health. Participants in the study were over 1,500 members of the Swedish police force. The study found that extensive organizational changes, such as downsizing or modification in work tasks, were associated with some increase in stress, disturbed sleep, incomplete recovery, and general health complaints; less extensive organizational changes, such as relocation, did not appear to be associated with the outcome variables. Perhaps the most compelling contribution of the study was the finding that *anticipation* of extensive organizational changes had nearly the same outcome as the actual changes, including association between sleep/work stress and depressive symptoms and gastrointestinal complaints. Information on the correlations between mental health and biological health may contribute to treatment approaches, with greater attention to the cognitive element of health threats.

*Police Style, Judgment, and Individual Well-Being.* Researchers Ilkka Salo and Carl Martin Allwood (2011) conducted a study of Swedish police investigators to analyze relationships between decision-making styles, judgmental self-doubt, and work-place conditions on the one hand and stress, quality of sleep, and burnout tendencies on the other. Measurement scales used by the researchers were classified as Judgmental Self Doubt, General Decision-Making, Satisfaction with Life, Performance-Based Self-Esteem, and Perceived Stress. The researchers also considered factors relating to work conditions and sleep quality. The study found correlations among non-decisiveness, high stress, and poor sleep. It also determined that self-worth and a tendency to avoid decision-making appear to be inversely related, and a high degree of correlation was found between stress and dependency in decision-making. Gender analyses revealed that male investigators exhibited higher values in rational decision-making style while female investigators sowed higher values in the dependent decision-making style. Female investigators also evidenced a higher degree of stress and performance-based self-esteem. The researchers pointed out that all participants in the study were from Swedish agencies and that the findings might not be fully applicable in police institutions in other countries. The work provides linkage between individual working style and outcomes and it suggests a need for individualized training programs to reduce stress and burnout. Understandings, preventions, and treatments do not appear to fashion themselves into a template solution. While the research corroborates the assertion that police people are individuals and require individual considerations in terms of their protection, health, and individualized versions of success, it also suggests that non-traditional characteristics of police health and well-being are important considerations.

*Special-Assignment Officers: Stress and Type of Work.* A recent thrust in law enforcement research has been to consider stress

24

in relation to specific law-enforcement assignments and special tactical deployment. Research by Garbarino, et al. (2012b) sought to evaluate stress levels among members of a specialized Italian police unit deployed for riot and crowd control. Protocols included before, during, and after psychological assessment questionnaires as well as other measures in integration. The study found that type-of-work was related to alterations in resilience and that members of the specialized unit had strong capacity to withstand stress. The study suggested that routine work may be more stressful for certain kinds of officers than assignment to special high-risk situations when adequate training and positive psychological support were provided. The cultural profile of an agency, or division within an agency, and individual personality traits may also be important factors. Thus, research by Garbarino, et al. (2012a) looked at individual personality profiles among Italian special force officers, finding that two thirds of the study group showed personality profiles similar to the general population, with the exception of higher self-reported emotional stability and self-deceptive enhancement. Nearly one third of test participants showed high emotive stability and organizational resilience scores, with low scores for anxiety, professional fatigue, callousness, and loss of empathy.

*Police Officers and Disabilities.* Police leaders benefit from information on individuals within their agency; likewise, individuals benefit from individualized consideration. Work by Dr. John Violanti (2012) was concerned with police officers with disabilities, pointing out that there are disabling factors in both acute and chronic stress which may contribute to perceptions of peer antagonism, may detract from a sense of control, and may create safety vulnerability. Feelings of clarity, power, and repute are diminished when disabled officers are, or believe they are, marginalized. Without respect, officers with disabilities may become outsiders—a perception that will likely worsen their conditions. Perhaps a most heroic step for officers is to seek help.

*Retention of Peace Officers.* Correlations between resilience, stress, and job satisfaction/dissatisfaction were highlighted in research by Criminal Justice Professor Eric G. Lambert (2007) and Lambert & Hogan (2006) who maintained that the hidden costs of turnover, particularly in high sensitivity areas such as corrections work, are generally immensely underestimated. They examined officer retention in relation to individual personality and attitude and in conjunction with situational, demographic, and environmental factors. Specific variables were job satisfaction, turnover intent, demographic characteristics, and work environment. Findings revealed that job satisfaction was the most significant factor effecting work environment; the work environment was the key variable in effecting intent to leave the job.

*Work, Status, and Job Satisfaction.* An impressive body of research has identified strong associations between work and health and has revealed that occupational stress can have positive or negative influences on the well-being of employees in any workplace, regardless of the size of the company, field of activity, or form of employment relationship. Researchers Romana Pasca & Shannon Wagner (2011) conducted studies in a multi-cultural Canadian workplace to examine occupational stress, mental health, and satisfaction as experienced by immigrant individuals attempting to achieve integration into Canadian workplaces. Participants were Canadian-born (CB) employees and nonCanadian-born employees (NCB) working in the fields of education, healthcare and/or social work. The researchers hypothesized that the level of occupational stress self-reported by NCB employees would be higher than the level self-reported by CB employees and that the NCB employees would have a lower level of perceived job satisfaction, life satisfaction, and marital satisfaction, and have more mental health issues than their CB counterparts. The authors utilized four measurement surveys: Satisfaction with Life Scale survey, Measure of Mental Health, the Symptom Checklist-90-Revised, and a Job Satisfaction Survey. The work revealed more similarities than differences between the two groups in the level of perceived occupational stress and suggested that achieving socio-professional status in the fields studied was a buffer against work-related stress.

Professor Jon M. Shane (2010) studied stress factors in police operations as well as organizationally embedded structural arrangements, policies, and practices. A former police captain, Professor Shane worked with data from two large urban police agencies and found distinct differences between operational and organizational stressors with a causal link between stress and performance. Moreover, he found that police organizations may contain contaminating elements that contribute to officer stress levels and actually diminish performance. Professor Shane recommended future similar studies of mid-size, suburban, and rural police agencies and the inclusion of superior officers and civilian police personnel.

In a book about emotional survival for peace officers, Professor Kevin M. Gilmartin (2002) describes a process in which a new police recruit may move from fresh and idealistic attitudes and perceptions to dark cynicism, callousness, fatigue, isolation, apathy, detachment, and anger. The dynamics of the deterioration process may in fact lead to self-destructive behavior patterns and, in some cases, to criminal behavior and degradation of meaning and value in a police person's life. Professor Gilmartin is a behavioral scientist and a former member of the Tucson, Arizona law enforcement agency; his book on emotional survival was intended to assist police officers and their families in addressing issues, improving quality of life, and remaining engaged in positive law-enforcement careers.

# Pressures Associated with Unethical Conduct

James E. Konopasek

What are the health and quality-of-life ramifications of unethical behavior for peace officers? What causes a clean cop to go dirty? How can a good officer prevent succumbing to pressures correlated with illegal, unethical, corrupt, and immoral behavior? Some insights are offered by Dr. James E. Konopasek, a polygraph examiner "too often" hired by police union attorneys to do "damage control" for officers facing employment termination.

Case examples of polygraph examinations conducted on police officers as a form of after-the-fact integrity testing (Tawny, 2008; Westen, 2010) tell the story. The first case is a big-city officer accused of sexually groping and photographing an under-the-influence female subject during a traffic stop. A second case example is a deputy working in a county jail initiating a sexual relationship with a female inmate inside the walls and continuing to engage in sexual relations after the inmate is released pending trial. Another case example is a small town officer accused of dealing thousands of dollars in steroids to a number of fellow officers. And yet another is a ten-year veteran accused of molesting his stepdaughter. As one police chief once stated with respect to officer misconduct, "it usually boils down to three things: money, drugs and sex."

During polygraph examinations on these individuals, pretest interviews revealed common threads: 1) all were deemed fit to be hired (passing paper/pencil tests, background checks, pre-employment polygraph exams, psychological tests) to the difficult job of a police officer; 2) all had served their communities for several years with good performance reviews; 3) none had ever been in disciplinary trouble before; and 4) all had recently experienced relationship, mood disorder, and financial problems.

A final, rather grim, commonality was present in this small group: all were *guilty* of unlawful, unprofessional, unethical conduct and were fired from their positions or pressured to resign. Whereas the dynamics of four cases do not provide anything more than anecdotal information, the experiences of four officers – coupled with some empirical evidence in the literature – provide insights on a problem that may cost police departments thousands of dollars and amass immeasurable human costs to the individuals involved.

Professor Ronald Akers's criminological social learning theory - SLT (Akers, 2009) offers a framework to address the question of what may cause an officer to become corrupt. Briefly, Akers postulates that four variables — imitation/modeling, differential association, definitions favorable to deviant behavior (attitudes and cognitions) and differential reinforcement—cause antisocial and prosocial behavior. The direction of behavior (prosocial/antisocial, legal/illegal, nondeviant/deviant, ethical/unethical) is determined by the degree, frequency, quality, and power of exposure the individual has to antisocial influences. For example, a new recruit, exposed on a daily basis to an upstanding, ethical field officer (who is a good role model, who associates with good coworkers and friends, who expresses by-the-book prosocial attitudes, and who reinforces the trainee with praise for good decisions and behavior) will likely be imitated. The reverse situation of corruptive influences being delivered by a superior officer will likely play out with the new recruit modeling unethical, and perhaps criminal, behaviors. In polygraph testing of the officers described above, direct imitation of poor behavior was not present; however, an organizational culture in which the afflicted and fellow officers minded their own business, looked the other way, failed to inquire, and simply "did not talk about it" appeared to be present.

The literature on unethical and corrupt criminal-justice system personnel is fairly limited. Pat A. Wertheim (1998), in the context of examining latent fingerprint examiners, speaks to the development of a "superiority complex," arrogance, diminished value of integrity expressed in mission statements, and erosion of department pride as factors contributing to fabrication of latent-print evidence. Marquart, Barnhill & Balshaw-Biddle (2001), studied 428 corrections officers working in Texas prisons who became engaged in unethical and illegal behavior. Termed "breaking custodial frame," boundary violations, or dual relationships, the disciplined (in various ways from verbal reprimand to termination) officers engaged in varying degrees of sexual conduct with inmates. Finding that approximately 80 per cent of sexual violators were female staff involved with male inmates, this research team determined that dual or overlapping relationships generally began with the following behaviors: exchanged glances, notes, photographs, rings, friendly smiles, and frequent conversations. The relationships were typified by "lovesickness" in which employees first became infatuated and then fell in love with inmates.

Of additional interest is the finding that in many cases supervisors knew of the relationships and practiced "willful blindness" to avoid scandal and embarrassment to the agency. Law Professor David Dorfman (1999) speaks to a similar cultural phenomenon describing the "wink and nod" of judges who may regularly accept incredible police testimony in the courtroom.

More prevalent with the officers described above was the presence of distorted thinking such as minimizing the illegal/unethical behavior, justifying wrongful acts or claiming circumstances beyond one's control as excuses for poor behavior. These factors relate to what criminologist Ronald Akers (2009) referred to as *definitions favorable to deviant behavior.* How a good officer begins to redefine his or her world — making minor transgressions acceptable or justified – is a critical turning point. Faulty thinking and antisocial attitudes greases the slope toward perpetration of more egregious illegal behaviors. In the case example of the steroid dealer, he then began to associate regularly with individuals who shared the view that buying/selling drugs was acceptable to give them an edge over "the truly bad guys" they were arresting on a daily basis (differential association and reinforcement – see Akers, 2009). In the sex-related case examples, different dynamics of differential association and reinforcement seemed to be in play including: excitement and positive feelings associated with excessive and/or illegal pornography use; positive emotions associated with sexual attention from a "taboo" and increased sense of power in personal life.

*Recommendations for Officers Facing Ethical Dilemmas.* From the above case examples provided, Dr. Konopasek makes the following recommendations for peace officers.

1. Remember that there is little more damaging to our profession – or more heart-wrenching to the humans involved — than to see a good cop gone bad;
2. Crooked cops are usually made through social learning processes;
3. Akers's criminological social learning theory (SLT) containing the crucial variables of imitation/modeling, definitions, differential association, differential reinforcement offers a framework for viewing how unethical behavior occurs and how such behavior may be corrected;
4. In line with SLT, be mindful of the behavior superiors are modeling – *imitate* prosocial, ethical, legal, and professional conduct;
5. Consistent with SLT, *associate* frequently with colleagues who maintain utmost professionalism and impeccable ethical standards – dissociate with those who do not;
6. Congruent with SLT, check yourself regarding how you are defining your world, your thinking, and your attitude (i.e., *definitions* favorable to law violation or unethical conduct).
7. Ask yourself, am I lying about, making excuses for, minimizing, rationalizing, or justifying poor behavior?
8. In line with SLT, expose yourself to influences that *differentially reinforce* good, ethical behavior;
9. Always be mindful of agency mission statements, codes of conduct, and ethics governing the police profession;
10. Discuss ethical dilemmas and avoid all behavior that could lead to your termination from the profession;
11. Avoid developing a "superiority complex," and distorted cognitions of "being above the law;"
12. Be mindful of organizational re-enforcers of ethical behavior.

> . . . Two roads diverged in a wood, and I –
> I took the one less traveled by,
> And that has made all the difference.

Robert Frost, *The Road Not Taken*

Among the many fruitful research contributions involving military veterans is a study by Yale University (School of Medicine) Professor R.H. Pietrzak et al. (2009) whose work was concerned with resilience and social support that may protect against PTSD. The researchers engaged 272 veterans and found that overall resilience scores were similar to those observed among civilian outpatient primary-care patients. Participants diagnosed with PTSD, however, were negatively associated with resilience measures of increased personal control and positive acceptance of change. The evidence strongly suggested that postdeployment support programs can serve as buffers against depressive and traumatic stress symptoms. All stress sufferers may benefit from proactive and preventative programs.

The conclusions by Professor Pietrzak and team are not at all surprising, and the Department of Veterans Administration (VA) has a number of postdeployment programs to assist veterans in their transition back to civilian life. Likewise, some law enforcement agencies have instituted support programs for veterans whose career paths take them into police work; in some cases, public-safety organizations have developed reactivation programs for veterans who are returning to law enforcement jobs after overseas military deployment. According to Police Captain Jeff Hink (Hink, 2010), as of November 2008, more than 120,000 members of the National Guard and military reserves were activated with roughly ten percent of the reservists being public-safety professionals. The Los Angeles County Sheriff's Department found that of its roughly 10,000 sworn personnel were 500 deployed reservists (since 2002). According to *GI Jobs.com,* a website for veterans seeking civilian employment, 80 percent of the Dallas Police Department's new hires over a two-year period were military vets; approximately 20 percent of Los Angeles Police Department officers have military backgrounds.

The transition from military service to law enforcement work is seldom routine, predictable, or smooth. According to Captain Hink's report on returning military veterans (Hink, 2010), more than one in four returning veterans will experience PTSD or other mental health issues; statistics from the VA suggest that the figure for veterans returning from Afghanistan and Iraq may be one in three. A portion of veterans returning to law enforcement jobs and a portion of law enforcement new hires may fall into this category.

31

Even more challenging and disheartening is the fact that a portion of returning veterans will come to the attention of law enforcement because of domestic violence or other criminal activity, homelessness, or substance abuse. Research developed by Major David Daniels of the United States Army School of Advanced Military examined correlations between PTSD and criminal behavior in soldiers who have been incarcerated after returning from the so-called Global War on Terror theaters (Daniels, 2008). The study used historical data from a number of sources, including the U.S. Bureau of Justice and the U.S. military disciplinary barracks to analyze historical trends in incarceration rates among veterans in federal and state correction facilities. The study revealed significant empirical data to support the probability that PTSD is a factor that influences veterans to commit violent acts leading to their eventual incarceration.

Daniels held that one can begin to make predictions regarding the effect this disorder will have on the military and their respective communities. Indeed, the title of his monograph was *Post-traumatic Stress Disorder and the Causal Link to Crime: A Looming National Tragedy.* He argued that our nation must come to fully appreciate the problem of PTSD and be proactive in our care for veterans before they become a domestic casualty of war.

Additional insight into the far-reaching issues concerning returning veterans is provided in a study by Professor Eric B. Elbogen and team (Elbogen et al., 2012) regarding financial difficulties experienced among veterans returning from Afghanistan and Iraq. Veterans who reported having money to cover basic needs were significantly less likely to have postdeployment adjustment problems such as criminal arrest, homelessness, substance abuse, suicidal behavior, and aggression. The study found that probable major depressive disorder, PTSD, and traumatic brain injury were associated with financial difficulties.

*Invisible Wounds.* The Hink (2010) report on returning military veterans revealed that 99 Army soldiers committed suicide in 2006. The report suggested that key factors in the decision to end their lives were failed relationships, legal and financial trouble, and job stress. While the wars in Iraq and Afghanistan have seen lower casualty rates of the killed or wounded than in earlier prolonged wars, it may be that invisible, unrecognized wounds are emerging as crucible for a different type of casualty. The report listed common factors leading to increased psychological stress in soldiers:

- Encountering roadside bombs, improvised explosive devices, and suicide bombers;
- Handling human remains;
- Killing an enemy;
- Seeing fellow soldiers and friends dead or injured;
- Experiencing helplessness.

An important work on "moral injury" (Litz et al., 2009) extended the list to include

- "perpetuating, failing to prevent, or bearing witness to acts that transgress deeply held moral beliefs and expectations."

The study acknowledged that military people have encountered moral and ethical dilemmas throughout history but held that research on the subject was sparse. The work was intended to provide a conceptual framework for examining the consequences of unnecessary acts of violence, for considering the lasting impact of morally injurious experiences, and for designing appropriate intervention strategies.

Commenting on the concept of "moral injury" and its repercussions, writer Tony Dokoupil (2012) made the statement that:

> . . . despite three decades of research and billions of dollars in government funding, America's servicemen and - women are not getting better. They are getting worse. Self-harm is now the leading cause of death for members of the Army, which has seen its suicide rate double since 2004, peaking this past summer with 38 in July alone. But the risk to discharged veterans may be even greater. Every month nearly 1,000 of them attempt to take their own lives. That's more than three attempts every 90 minutes, at least one of them successful. (Dokoupil, 2012).

The writer further commented that military people are

> . . . shuttling between two worlds: ours, where thou shalt not kill is chiseled into everyday life, and another, where thou better kill, be killed, or suffer the shame of not trying. There is no more hellish commute.

Dokoupil related that one of the researchers in the Litz study, Shira Maguen, found in clinical studies that killing in combat doubled the risk of suicidal thinking among Vietnam veterans; among Iraq veterans she found that the act of killing predicted not only PTSD but also alcohol abuse, marital problems, and anger management issues.

Dukoupil observed that a new definition of PTSD may be in the making, a definition that shifts focus away from what others do to soldiers onto what they, themselves, do to others, or in some cases fail to do *for* each other. Clearly a new definition will need to plumb the depths of shame and soul-tearing sorrow. The fact of war itself, regardless of its moral or ethical justifications, may also be up for reconsideration. Moral damage is not an affliction suffered exclusively by veterans. As powerfully argued in Lieutenant Colonel Dave Grossman's book, *On Killing: The Psychological Cost of Learning to Kill in War and Society* (Grossman, 2009), " The psychological cost for soldiers . . . is devastating. The psychological cost for the rest of us is even greater: Contemporary civilian society, particularly the media, replicates the army's conditioning techniques and directly contributes to our rising rate of violent crime, especially among the young.

# Mounting Pressures – Is There a Cavalry on the Way?

It is not the intent of this work to suggest specific medical treatments for diseases related to high-stress occupations. Health-care professionals have deep concern, vast amounts of information, and sound advice for individuals who suffer from stress-related afflictions. That said, we are nevertheless concerned with assisting readers in understanding the nature of stressors in order to consider reliable individual life-style changes and societal prevention and mitigation measures. There are many new and promising methods and approaches that can be helpful in the pursuit of police health, whether preventative, restorative, or, optimally, proactive.

## The Institute of Heart Math and "The Coherent Heart" : New Directions in Psychophysiological Stress Management

For a number of years, researchers at The Institute of HeartMath have been developing and refining technologies and treatment for individuals engaged in high-stress occupations. Indeed, police officers and military personnel have taken part in a number of the research studies and in the resulting programs aimed at proactively supporting mental health and providing tools for dealing with stressor events as they happen. The term "coherence" is used by the institute to describe a healthful state of balance that supports *mental, physical, spiritual, and emotional* well being. A HeartMath program called "The Coherence Advantage" encompasses the notion that what we consider negative emotions – anger, worry, resentment, insecurity, self-doubt, anxiety, impatience, etc. – are in fact disruptors of optimal physical body and mental functions. They drain energy; they release stress hormones; they disrupt the body's brain and nervous system; and they diminish the power of the body's healing processes. In contrast, emotions we consider positive do literally facilitate healthful physiological functions, renew energy, optimize the body's communicative and regenerative processes, offer respite from the toxicity of stress reactions, and support efficiency in the body's interactive systems.

Understanding the term "coherence" is a first step in addressing stress-related challenges and afflictions. The coherent state may also be called a "heart-focused" and positive condition. In a broad sense, coherence simply suggests a state of being logically integrated, consistent, and intelligible; different parts of a system work together in harmony and consistency, with an efficient use of energy. Thus, the whole is greater than the sum of its parts (Bradley, McCraty, Lash, & Laraway, 2011). Imagine, for example, hearing individual notes played randomly on a piano as opposed to hearing a well-known symphonic composition played by a full concert orchestra. Now imagine the vast array of rhythmic activities of the human body at any moment as it receives and processes simultaneous signals such as waves of sound and pressure in biophysiological terms, hormonal and neurotransmissions, biochemical flows, neural impulses, and interactions within the body's electromagnetic fields. The brain and the heart are in constant communication, with the brain serving as highly efficient data processor but with the heart serving as the rhythmic conductor for the whole. The brain, in all its glory, barely produces one five thousandth of the electromagnetic field that the heart does! Additionally, the heart's emanations can pass right through body tissues and out into the external world as well. Magnometers can gauge the heart's emanating fields with ease and accuracy. Thus, feeling another or sensing the presence of another is not only plausible but measurable. These energetic field interactions can be considered separately from symbols and other communications that are spoken, for example, and are quite plainly readable. Recent and remarkable studies by the Institute also show a relationship between the heart and intuitive processes, suggesting the heart participates in receiving, processing, and decoding intuitive information before the brain does.

HeartMath programs acknowledge that the degree of coherence in individual thoughts, feelings, and social interactions may vary widely from moment to moment, day to day. For that reason, the programs and technologies emphasize techniques for building resilience capacity with an understanding that interconnectedness and coherence are keys to human resilience. HeartMath tools may be used before, during, and after traumatic or stressful situations to assist in regulating the body's naturally healthy flow. Organizations that have used the coherence practice tools have found that the benefits of training extend over longer and longer time periods as participants continue to engage in the training regimen and possibly attain an ability to develop autocoherence wherein benefits of training remain fairly constant and result in a state of sustained high coherence. The following chart shows the intended and achievable outcomes of HeartMath coherence and resilience training and practice.

## Coherence Training Outcomes

- Enhanced performance
- Understanding of resilience: What drains it and renews it
- Improved decision-making in complex environments
- Improved situational self- awareness
- Breathing coherence, for reducing the intensity of stress reactions
- Reestablishing self control through Shift and Reset™ training
- Preparation for challenging situations
- Establishment of a coherent baseline for sustaining resilience and emotional flexibility
- Enhanced awareness of others, for building unit cohesion
- Provision for ongoing institutional reinforcement through peer- and superior-officer mentoring

Source: Institute of HeartMath

As we have seen in previous pages of this work, operational stress on police officers can have *accumulated* deleterious effects. In a HeartMath study involving police officers, researchers determined that coherence activation and use significantly affected outcomes in police performance. Cooperative engagements were increased while incidences of competiveness and dysfunction were marginalized *and* diminished. Police participants in the study reported and demonstrated higher levels of patience, understanding, and ability to reflect critically. The research further uncovered potentials for improved team listening and communication as well as for increased caring and compassion. The following chart statistically reveals some of the improvements from the HeartMath Coherence Advantage training for police officers.

## Police Coherence Advantage

- Improves ability to manage moods (83%)
- Improves capacity to listen patiently to family members and be understanding of their concerns (75%)
- Enables greater individual insight into psychological well-being (58%)
- Improves ability to integrate intuition into actions at work (8%)
- Improves tendency to discuss personal life matters with co-workers (8%)
- Improves tendency to discuss with co-workers emotionally difficult situations encountered on the job (17%)

Source: The Institute of HeartMath

In the assessment phase of the HeartMath Coherence Advantage training for police officers, researchers found the following outcomes:

- Decreased stress symptoms
- Increased positive emotions, peacefulness, and vitality
- Decreased sleeplessness, indigestion, and anxiety

Perhaps the most rewarding outcome for participants in Coherence Advantage training is gaining awareness that individuals' own perceptions are likely to be the major contributors to stressful or calm moments in their lives. We have previously used the firetruck siren as an example. It is apt to be a stressor for pedestrians, but a useful tool for the fireman driver; a waterfall in a mountain stream may be serene and calming for one individual but fear-inducing for another. Once an individual acknowledges that s/he is the most important participant in recovery from stress-induced afflictions, there is frequently a sense of new freedom and hope. No longer a hostage of past experiences, the individual may very quickly experience added clarity, ability to focus, and ability to develop calmness under pressure.

The idea that positive emotions and elevated states of consciousness can support positive transformation has been around for hundreds, indeed perhaps thousands of years. Until quite recently, however, there has been little reliable scientific work to explore the actual bodily functions, mechanisms, and patterns related to elevated states. The research by the Institute of Heart Math has clearly shown that positive emotions and health are linearly related in outcomes; in addition, there appears to be a strong correlations between positive emotive health and creativity, problem solving and innovation, cognitive plasticity, and a lowering of learning resistance.

Coherence training is supported by an Institute of HeartMath device called an emWave. This easy-to-use tool allows the user to observe, minute-by-minute, the results of his/her efforts to transform stress reactions into improved wellness and enhanced personal growth. Practice with this coherence regimen supports an increasing ability to seek recalibration of the phychophysiological system even, or perhaps especially, while under duress. The emWave tool collects pulse data and translates the information from heart rhythms into graphics that help users change their heart rhythm patterns in order to create coherence – now known to be a scientifically measurable condition characterized by harmony in both psychological and physiological processes. (Please see Section III, page 71, for further discussion of HeartMath innovations, especially the Global Coherence Initiative.

**The Institute of HeartMath** is located at
14700 West Park Avenue,
Boulder Creek, CA 95006
Telephone: (831) 338-8500 or (800) 711-6221
Email: info@heartmath.org

**The extensive research library of the Institute may be accessed at www.heartmath.org/research/research-home/research-center-home.html**

*HeartMath and Organizational Advantages.* HeartMath programs relating to heart-centered consciousness have offered stress-management tools for peace officers for a number of years in organizational settings. One research program was centered on correctional officers in California and was funded in part by POST (McCraty, et al., 2009). Correctional officers may be routinely exposed to cognitive dissonance stress factors beyond the range of normal conditions, factors such as altercations, confrontations, sporadic violence, negative emotions relating to hopelessness and despair, shift-work disruptions of the sleep cycle, authoritarian and/or threat-based cultures, planning conflicts, lack of sturdy career efficacy, neglect of the human need to achieve, and other aspects of workplace stressors frequently researched in organizational psychology. The test groups were given specialty training that was intended to improve individuals' emotional self-regulation and to mitigate the harmful effects of stress. The study revealed gains in officer motivation and productivity, perception of support, and clarity of purpose, while also revealing a recognizable decrease in health-treatment costs. The chart below displays some of factors revealed by the study wherein health-care costs and risks can be offset.

## Health Risk and Cost Factors

| *Factor* | *Risk/Cost Factor Yes / No - %* |
|---|---|
| **Depression** | YES – 70 |
| **Stress** | YES – 46 |
| **Blood Glucose** | YES – 35 |
| **Body Weight** | YES – 21 |
| **Blood Pressure** | YES – 12 |
| **Inactivity** | YES – 10 |

**Source:** McCraty, Atkinson, Lipsenthal, and Arguelles, 2009.

## Mindsight

A graduate of Harvard Medical School, a clinical professor of psychiatry, a mental-health pioneer, and a visionary healer of more than 25 years, Dr. Daniel J. Siegel has written extensively about our human capability to heal. Opportunities for positive change are enhanced by practices that consider the brain to be re-wireable rather than hard-wired for a single pattern. Mindsight programs and practices focus internally on certain mental processes in such a way that individuals have the opportunity to alter their ordinary neural networking habits. Siegel's work merges psychotherapeutic practice with brain science to examine the interface of human relationships and basic biological processes, creating a basis for integrating and bolstering natural self-healing and achievement of well-being. Transformative mindfulness processes may include examining past and/or irrational fears and controlling emotions such as anger, escaping self-destructive cycles and addictive or mindlessly habituated behaviors, releasing conflict patterns, cultivating intuitive listening regarding the body and its signaling procedures, mastering emotions, and healing relationships. In short, mindfulness is about our ability to re-sculpt our neural pathways and thus to consciously and intentionally transform our lives (Siegel, 2010). A particular strength of the Mindsight programs is the success it has enjoyed in treating PTSD and other internal pains.

Dr. Siegel argues that human beings need to be "cognitively mindful"; that is, our minds must be available for new contexts, must be able to observe subtlety, to take on novelty in perceptive in-feeds, and to examine events in the current, absent from historical categorization. The desired state of being involves a hemispheric crossover between left and right brain function and allows adaptive, coherent, highly flexible, energized and yet stable psychoemotive balance in the mind. In a mindfully aware state, a person does not access learning and memory directly, but uses overlap of those categories to bridge cognition and affect, thought, and feeling. Layers of well-bring and resilience are included in the process of mindful learning, for example, where the experiences of currency, novelty, and discernment are used to shape the color and enjoyment of a heightened learning capability. Actions that adorn the theoretical premise of mindfulness in Dr. Siegel's work include putting the classification process on hold, emancipating new information from old cortical processes, reflecting consciously in the present, and binding ancient wisdoms with neural insights and clinical practice. In building reflective practice, the process of attunement can be extremely useful, particularly in modeling and teaching situations.

Dr. Siegel (2010) asserts that many prevalent cultures in the world are in some ways "broken" and require a fix that rediscovers harmony in life. The mindfulness practice may be considered a means of harnessing the brain in the cultivation of well-being. By brightening the conscious mind and awareness, individuals may take significant steps toward overcoming the imprisonment of past experiences. An important first step is to cultivate understanding of the core self, not simply the social self, and to embrace the neurobiology of care, of uncertainty, and of mortality.

In addition to academic research publications, Dr. Siegel has published widely for professionals and for individuals and families.

---

*The Developing Mind: How Relationships and the Brain Interact to Shape Who We Are* (2012, revised edition).

*The Mindful Brain: Reflection and Attunement in the Cultivation of Well-Being* (2007)

*The Mindful Therapist: A Clinician's Guide to Mindsight and Neural Integration* (2012)

*Pocket Guide to Interpersonal Neurobiology: An Integrative Handbook of the Mind* (2012).

*Mindsight: The New Science of Personal Transformation* (2010)

*Parenting from the Inside Out: How a Deeper Self-Understanding Can Help You Raise Children Who Thrive* (2003) with Mary Hartzell

*The Whole-Brain Child: 12 Revolutionary Strategies to Nurture Your Child's Developing Mind* (2011)

Dr. Siegel is co founder of the UCLA Mindful Awareness Research Center. http://marc.ucla.edu/

---

***Mindfulness, Meditation, and Stress Reduction.*** As early as 1992 and under the direction of Professor of Medicine Jon Kabat-Zinn, researchers at University of Massachusetts Medical School (Kabat-Zinn et al., 1992) attempted to determine if meditation could reduce symptoms of anxiety disorders. They found that *group* mindfulness meditation training programs were effective in reducing such symptoms, including agoraphobia, and in improving relaxation. In a later study (Speca, Carlson, Goodey, & Angen, 2000), researchers attempted to determine the effects of mindfulness-based meditation as a tool for stress reduction and mood balancing. Participants in the study were cancer patients — male and female patients with a wide variety of cancer diagnoses, stages of illness, and ages.

Special attention was paid to the issues of anxiety, depression, confusion, and anger. Benefits from the group mindfulness meditation program ranged from simple stress reduction to modifications of biochemical, physiological, and psychological aspects. Mood disturbance was lowered by 65 percent, with a 31 percent reduction in symptoms of stress. The exercises involved reflecting on mind-body as well as changing habituation patterns from destructive and harmful ones that induce stress to healthy ones that can be harbingers of new cognitive and rational-emotive balance and freedoms as well as healthy neurochemical flow.

Within a few years, there were numerous studies involving structured group programs aimed at reducing suffering from physical, psychosomatic, and psychiatric disorders by way of mindfulness-based meditation.. A research team at Freiburg Institute for Mindfulness Research, Freiburg, Germany (Grossman, et al., 2004) conducted a meta-analysis of nonreligious and nonesoteric programs that offered systematic procedures to support enhanced awareness of moment-by-moment experiences and mental processes. Particular attention was given to anxiety, depression, heart disease, and cancer as well as some non-clinical issues. The study concluded that *a broad range of individuals* may benefit from mindfulness-based program, and within the last few years, there has been a wealth of studies focusing on specific diseases and conditions as well as new technological advances in measuring the effects of mindfulness-based meditation and training.

One of the treasures that has emerged from mindfulness research in recent years is a collaborative work by Professors Kabat-Zinn and Richard Davidson who served as editors of *The Mind's Own Physician: A Scientific Dialogue with the Dalai Lama on the Healing Power of Meditation* (Kabat-Zinn & Davidson, 2012). The work is the most recent in a series initiated by the Mind and Life Institute which brings the Dalai Lama together with leading researchers in medicine, psychology, and neuroscience to explore the healing potential of the human mind. The Institute also sponsored the publication of an earlier work on *The Science and Clinical Applications of Meditation* (website: www.mindandlife.org). Please see page 72 for a list of other Mind and Life Institute publications and some of the Dalai Lama's most recent works.

A partial list of additional mindfulness research within the last few years follows. Readers who wish to access these studies via the Internet may enter the title of the article in a search engine, or if a doi number is listed, simply enter the number.

Self-directed Mindfulness Training and Improvement in Blood Pressure, Migraine Frequency, and Quality of Life. *Global Advances in Health and Medicine (*2013), *2(2)*20-25.

Mindfulness Starts with the Body: Somatosensory Attention and Top-down Modulation of Cortical Alpha Rhythms in Mindfulness Meditation. *Frontiers in Human Neuroscience* (2013). doi: 10.3389/fnhum.2013.00012.

Brain Changes in Long-term Zen Meditators Using Proton Magnetic Resonance Spectroscopy and Diffusion Tensor Imaging: *PLoS One.* (2013). doi: 10.1371/journal.pone.0058476

Neural Mechanisms of Attentional Control in Mindfulness Meditation. *Frontiers in Neuroscience* (2013). doi: 10.3389/fnins.2013.00008.

Mindfulness-based Cognitive Behavior Therapy in Patients with Anxiety Disorders. *Indian Journal of Psych9ological Medicine* ( 2012) 34(3), 263-9. doi: 10.4103/0253-7176.106026

An Update on Mindfulness Meditation as a Self-help Treatment for Anxiety and Depression. *Psychology Research and Behavior Management.* National Institutes of Health (2012) doi: 10.2147/PRBM.S34937

Effects of Mindful-attention and Compassion Meditation Training on Amygdala Response to Emotional Stimuli in an Ordinary, Non-meditative State. *Frontiers in Human Neuroscience.*(2012). doi: 10.3389/fnhum.2012.00292.

The Effects of Mindfulness-based Cognitive Therapy on Affective Memory Recall Dynamics in Depression. *Frontiers in Human Neuroscience.* (2012). doi: 10.3389/fnhum.2012.00257.

Complementary Medicine, Exercise, Meditation, Diet, and Lifestyle Modification for Anxiety Disorders: A Review of Current Evidence. *Evidence-Based Complementary and Alternative Medicine* (2012) doi:10.1155/2012/809653

Is it Me or Not Me? Modulation of Perceptual-motor Awareness and Visuomotor Performance by Mindfulness Meditation. *BMC Neuroscience* (2012) doi: 10.1186/1471-2202-13-88.

Mindfulness Online: A Preliminary Evaluation of the Feasibility of a Web-based Mindfulness Course and the Impact on Stress. *BMJ Open* (2012) doi 10.1136/bmjopen-2011-000803

Hypertension Analysis of Stress Reduction Using Mindfulness Meditation and Yoga (The HARMONY Study). *BMJ Open* ( 2012) doi: 10.1136/bmjopen-2012-000848

**Regular, Brief Mindfulness Meditation Practice Improves Electrophysiological Markers of Attentional Control.** *Frontiers of Human Neuroscience* (2012). doi: 10.3389/fnhum.2012.00018

**Mindfulness Training Alters Emotional Memory Recall Compared to Active Controls: Support for an Emotional Information Processing Model of Mindfulness.** *Frontiers of Human Neuroscience* (2012). doi: 10.3389/fnhum.2012.00015

**The Validation of an Active Control Intervention for Mindfulness Based Stress Reduction (MBSR).** *Behavior Research and Therapy* (2012) doi: 10.1016/j.brat.2011.10.011

**Mindfulness-based Stress Reduction for Patients with Anxiety Disorders.** *Behaviour Research and Therapy* (2011). doi: 10.1016/jbrat.2011.01.007

**Mindful Awareness and Non-judging in Relation to Posttraumatic Stress Disorder Symptoms.** *Mindfulness (N Y)* (2011), 2(4), 219-227.

**Mindfulness-based Stress Reduction: A Non-pharmacological Approach for Chronic Illnesses.** *North American Journal of Medical Science* (2011). doi: 10.4297/najms.2011.320

**Mindfulness-based Stress Reduction for HIV Treatment Side Effects.** *Journal of Pain and Symptom Management* (2012) doi: 10.1016/j.jpainsymman.2011.04.007

**Loving-kindness and Compassion Meditation: Potential for Psychological Interventions.** *Clinical Psychology Review* (2011). doi: 10.1016/j.cpr.2011.07.003.

**A Randomized, Controlled Trial of Meditation for Work Stress, Anxiety and Depressed Mood in Full-time Workers.** *Evidence-Based Complementary and Alternative Medicine* (2011) doi: 10.1155/2011/960583

**Dialectics of Mindfulness: Implications for Western Medicine.** *Philosophy, Ethics, and Humanities in Medicine* (2011). doi:10.1186/1747-5341-6-10

**Brain Mechanisms Supporting the Modulation of Pain by Mindfulness Meditation.** *Journal of Neuroscience* (2011) doi: 10.1523/JNEUROSCI.5791-10.2011

**Mindfulness-based Stress Reduction Versus Pharmacotherapy for Chronic Primary Insomnia.** *Explore (NY)* (2011). doi: 10.1016/j.explore.2010.12.003

**Changes in Spirituality Partly Explain Health-related Quality of Life Outcomes after Mindfulness-Based Stress Reduction.** *Journal of Behavioral Medicine* (2011). doi: 10.1007/s10865-011-9332-x.

**Mindfulness Practice Leads to Increases in Regional Brain Gray Matter Density.** *Psychiatry Research* (2011). doi: 10.1016/j.pscychresns.2010.08.006.

Much of the early work done by Professor of Medicine Jon Kabat-Zinn formed the framework for today's successful mindfulness-based stress reduction programs in medical centers and health maintenance organizations throughout the country. Professor Kabat-Zinn was a student of Buddhist teachers, and his studies encouraged him to integrate those teachings with Western medical practice concerned with stress, pain, and illness. In addition to numerous scientific studies, Professor Kabat-Zinn is author of the following works:

---

*Full Catastrophe Living: Using the Wisdom of Your Body and Mind to Face Stress, Pain, and Illness* (1991)

*Wherever You Go, There You Are: Mindfulness Meditation in Everyday Life* (1994)

*Full Catastrophe Living: How to Cope with Stress, Pain and Illness Using Mindfulness Meditation* (1996)

*The Power of Meditation and Prayer*, with Sogyal Rinpoche, Larry Dossey, Michael Toms (1997)

*Everyday Blessings: The Inner Work of Mindful Parenting*, with Myla Kabat-Zinn (1997)

*Mindfulness Meditation for Everyday Life* (2001)

*Wherever You Go, There You Are: Mindfulness Meditation in Everyday Life* (2005)

*Coming to Our Senses: Healing Ourselves and the World Through Mindfulness* (2006)

*The Mindful Way Through Depression: Freeing Yourself from Chronic Unhappiness* with J. Mark G. Williams, John D. Teasdale and Zindel V. Segal (2007)

*Arriving at Your Own Door* (2008)

*Letting Everything Become Your Teacher: 100 Lessons in Mindfulness* (2009)

*The Mind's Own Physician: A Scientific Dialogue with the Dalai Lama on the Healing Power of Meditation*, with Richard Davidson (2012)

Professor Kabat-Zinn is a board member of the Mind and Life Institute which organizes dialogues between the Dalai Lama and Western scientists.

---

Mindfulness-based stress reduction is intended to help participants become more aware of thoughts, body sensations, and feelings and to cultivate discerning observations of the various stimuli that enter their awareness. Participants gain in ability to cogently develop meaning as opposed to drawing continuously from old belief systems that can contaminate new experiences; they learn to let go of past disabling events and fears about the future, to heighten quality-of-life considerations, and to increase compassion for themselves and others. Successful clinical applications of mindfulness practice are evident in PTSD treatments, in which patients/clients can experience, in the present moment, sensations and the body's varied awareness cues without re-experiencing traumas that may be associated mentally/emotionally with given experiences. Another benefit of mindfulness practice lies in the development of neural plasticity which is promoted by emotive engagement, novelty contextualization, attention arousal, and exercise. The coherent-mind state encourages and supports integrated neural function whether within a psychotherapeutic environment or simply in an individual's search for well-being through mindfulness practice. In the challenge of attaining left and right hemispheric balance and in overcoming resistances, interferences, and distracting barriers, there is promise of deep and visceral understanding of life that may be communicable by way of reflective functioning, as in mindfulness, reflective modeling, and perhaps neurolinguistic programming (Siegel, 2007; O'Connor & Seymour, 2011; Heal, 2012).

The evolving practice of *Neurolinguistic Programming* is another vigorous attempt in psychotherapy, personal transformation, and advanced communications to support a mindful learning process. While scientific validation lags, many practitioners use neurolinguistic programming in their communications medicine chests (O'Connor & Seymour, 2011; Heal, 2012). Various issues such as resistance to a mindful state, inattentiveness, habituated mental dysfunction, phobias, and depressions challenge fruitful awareness and communications. Neurolinguistic programming provides a method to minimize such distractions by acknowledging that invisible thought processes are made visible and interpretable by the body's accompanying physiological reactions. In a therapeutic setting, neurolinguistic programming focuses on desired outcome rather than on a presented problem. The process involves establishing rapport with listeners, obtaining information regarding agenda and bias, integrating change procedures, and developing tools for interventions. The process also engages state-of-mind assessment, non-verbal cue recognition mirroring, paced rehearsal, and meta-modeling (O'Connor & Seymour, 2011) in order to span perceptive levels and provide enhanced learning for the curious and dedicated. The process also respects the role of intuition in allowing decision-makers to quickly grasp the essence of a situation, sort through a vast amount of ambiguous and uncertain information, and find an acceptable resolution— a particularly useful tool for law enforcement personnel.

*Cognitive Behavior Therapy* is another program developed to assist patients in changing their patterned reactions to emotional stimuli. The therapist and patient work as a team to "reprogram" habituated responses and reduce patients' vulnerability to dysfunctional emotions and/or maladaptive behavior. The synergistic therapy may use a number of techniques to help individuals understand and challenge their behavior patterns and to diminish the impact of emotional distress and self-defeating responses. This form of therapy is problem focused and directed at helping patients develop specific action strategies to alleviate both symptoms and vulnerability. A useful introduction to Cognitive Behavior Therapy is available at the Internet website www.beckinstitute.org/what-is-cognitive-behavioral-therapy

*Re-evaluation Counseling (Peer Counseling)* is another therapeutic process whereby people of all backgrounds can learn to help one another address the effects of past accumulated distress experiences in an effort to free themselves of disabling emotions and behaviors. Participants learn to discharge emotions and to re-evaluate their experiences and their potential for healing behaviors and practices. An overview of the process and contact information is available at the website http://rc.org.

*Service Work and Mindsight.* It is perhaps ironic that healthcare professionals, police officers, and others whose work is involved in caring for others are among the individuals most frequently threatened by stress-related afflictions. A pilot study by Shapiro, Astin, Bishop, & Cordova (2005) resulted in a recommendation for an eight-week mindfulness-based stress-reduction program for healthcare workers. Such a program is applicable and available to law enforcement agencies and to police officers seeking to better sustain themselves. Some of the barriers to implementation are familiar: budget and time constraints and denial of need. Once distrust and denial of need are conquered, planners frequently turn to grant opportunities to instigate innovative programs.

Readers seeking to investigate or expand stress-reduction programs in their organizations may find useful information at the *Grantmakers for Effective Organizations* Internet website: www.geofunders.org/about. The term "widespread empathy" is used by the organization in discussing tool sets to support organizations in moving from chaos to success. The mission of many philanthropic organizations is frequently to counter forces of injustice, inequity, poverty, and ignorance by way of harmonious and mutually supportive operations among people in organizations. The grantmakers organization points out that innovations may provide tools for change but in order to be beneficial must also be accompanied by progressive discernment and mindfulness in which the individual level of empathy is scaled up into the organizational culture. Police officers who "work the streets" in support of a compassionate and empathetic society may accept the challenge of transferring insights and understanding into the organization.

Another useful website for individuals seeking stress-reduction tools is ***Lumosity's Human Cognition Project: www/hcp.lumosity.com***. Not everyone, not every organization, can commit to a full eight weeks of the mindfulness-based stress reduction, and the Luminosity site is designed to assist individuals in strengthening ability to ignore irrelevant stimuli and negative emotions while strengthening selective attention and working memory. The game-based training exercises have also been shown to have positive emotional benefits for individuals suffering from chronic pain, depression, and traumatic injuries.

## Well Being Theory and Positive Psychology

*Positive Psychology* is concerned with the scientific study of strengths and virtues that enable individuals and communities to flourish. Positive psychology focuses on promoting mental health rather than simply treating illness and has three central concerns: Positive emotions, positive individual traits, and positive institutions (Seligman & Csikszentmihalyi, 2000). Abraham Maslow, Carl Rogers, and Erich Fromm are among the humanist psychologists who developed theories and practices concerned with human happiness. Empirical support for some of their theories has recently been provided by Psychology Professor Martin Seligman who serves as the director of the Positive Psychology Center at University of Pennsylvania. The center supports and relates well-being research and provides educational programs as well as resources for teachers (http://www.ppc.sas.upenn.edu/).

Professor Seligman is the co-author with Psychology Professor Christopher Peterson of *Character Strength and Virtues: A Handbook and Classification (*2004) and is author of *Authentic Happiness* (2003) and *Flourish: A Visionary New Understanding of Happiness and Well-Being (2011)*. Professor Seligman's well-being theory, as described in his most recent book, consists of five measureable elements, highlighted by the acronym PERMA:

> **P**ositive emotions
> **E**ngagement
> **R**elationships and social connections
> **M**eaning
> **A**ccomplishment

Dr. Seligman points out that some elements of PERMA are measured subjectively by self-reporting, but others can be measured objectively. In all cases, he maintains,

> Well-being cannot exist just in your own head: well-being is a combination of feeling good as well as actually having meaning, good relationships, and accomplishment. The way we choose our course in life is to maximize all five of these elements. . . . Your highest strengths are deployed to meet the highest challenges that come your way (Seligman, 2011, Newsletter).

The United States Army has used Dr. Seligman's work extensively in its emotional resilience programs as have many major corporations that seek to heighten productivity and performance and to understand how they may do so by increasing their employees' well-being. The **Comprehensive Soldier Fitness Program** was introduced by the Army in 2009 in recognition of the stresses resulting from persistent conflicts and demands for high operational performance. It was considered a holistic fitness program intended to enhance performance and build resilience not only among soldiers but for families and Army civilians as well. The five specific elements of the program are: Physical performance, positive emotional balance, fulfilling social engagements, supportive and safe family interactions/resources; and spiritual strengths.

*How Positive Emotions Heal.* Research by Dr. Barbara Fredrickson, Kenan Distinguished Professor in the Department of Psychology, University of North Carolina, and director of the Positive Emotions and Psychophysiology Laboratory has fruitfully directed her research toward developing the ability to self-generate meaningful positive emotions; her **broaden-and-build theory** holds that positive emotions expand individuals' awareness and that these moments of awareness accumulate to increase opportunities for well-being. Her recent research data from multiple laboratories deepen evidence that contemplative practices transform biological functioning in ways that promote mental and physical health. Dr. Fredrickson recently presented her theory and supporting evidence at 2012 International Research Congress on Integrative Medicine and Health sponsored by the Consortium of Academic Health Centers for Integrative Medicine. Additional information is available at the website:imconsortium.org/.

## Integrative Health and Medicine/Mind-Body Connections

For those of us raised on polio vaccine, penicillin shots, and Neosporin, it may be a serious overload to consider the vast array of medical practices, mind-body therapies, nutritional supplements, herbal remedies, etc. that fill our e-mails and advertising supplements. What is homeopathy, naturopathy, Ayurveda; what are Qigong, Reiki, and electromagnetic therapy?

It did not always require a guru, sage, or mystical ascent leader to understand harmonies. For instance, with regard to nutrition, there are local products that are fresh, there are specific seasons for specific fresh products, and there are naturally fortifying ingredients in each product. But in our environment, there are also poisons, toxins, abuses and misuses. As we peel the proverbial onion, we can probably accept the notion that sleep may be the most restorative thing the mind-body does; good nutrition and exercise are vital. And we can ask some simple questions.

**How well are we sleeping?**

**What are we eating and breathing?**

**Are we creating many of the diseases that afflict us?**

This work will not attempt to investigate processed sugar, caffeine addiction, pesticides in our food, air quality in our cities, or genetically modified vegetable seeds in our gardens. But one must wonder if there would be a trillion-dollar healthcare empire in the United States if we had a thorough understanding of sleep, nutrition, and exercise embedded in our consciousness. Some philosophers, theologians, and medical practitioners argue that we do, indeed, have such information available, should we only learn to access it. In his book *Power vs. Force: The Hidden Determinants of Human Behavior*, Dr. David R. Hawkins, for example, argued that:

> Each of us possesses a computer far more advanced than the most elaborate artificial intelligence machine available, one that's available at any time — the human mind itself [through which] the body can discern, to the finest degree, the difference between that which is supportive of life and that which is not (Hawkins, 2012, p. 45).

Though not a immediately obvious part of mainstream healthcare notions, Dr. Hawkins' work provides readers with challenging and fascinating concepts that have been the subject of many lectures and demonstrations at some of the world's leading universities and religious centers. He maintained that consciousness and health are inevitably connected; that the body's responses shift from moment-to-moment as an outcome of an individual's thoughts and associated emotions; that habituated responses over time result in progressive change in patterns, and that the patterns eventually become apparent in sophisticated medical measuring tools such as electron microscopy, magnetic imaging, X-rays, etc.

"We could say," Dr. Hawkins wrote, "that the invisible universe of thought and attitude becomes visible as a consequence of the body's habitual response" (Hawkins, 2012, p. 218). It is certainly quite obvious that not all health concerns result from individual choice, thoughts, and attitudes, but it is a hope-giving awareness to understand that positive attitudes are associated with good health; negative emotions such as anxiety, hostility, and fear relate to disease.

The notion that the human body has within it an elaborate process for discerning life-destructive or life-supportive patterns is frequently reflected in integrative health and wellness programs. With notable spokesmen such as Deepak Chopra, Dr. Andrew Weil, and Prince Charles leading the march, the parade of integrated nutrition and integrated health practices that is energizing the country is aimed at integrating life's drills and requirements with life benefits, health and happiness to be achievable by way of spiritual practice, healthful diets, career and fitness decisions, love and relationships — all geared toward personal growth and well-being. Unfortunately, many approaches to the pursuit of good health do not fit with our insurance claims and are out of sync with profit-seeking enterprises that dominate the healthcare industry.

For readers who are interested in pursuing integrative health-care approaches, there are a number or organizations devoted to supporting evidence-based information and practices. Integrated nutrition and medicine need not be small concerns nor special interest niches, but rather valid paths of inquiry with tremendous potential. Some contact information is on the following page.

**Consortium of Academic Health Centers for Integrative Medicine**
D513 Mayo, Mail Code 505
420 Delaware Street SE
Minneapolis, MN 55455
612-624-9166 fax: 612-626-5280 .www.imconsortium.org/.

**Arizona Center for Integrative Medicine**
**University of Arizona**
P.O. Box 245153
Tucson, AZ 85724-5153
http://integrativemedicine.arizona.edu/about/

**National Center for Complementary and Alternative Medicine**
U.S. Department of Health and Human Services
National Institute of Health
31 Center Drive, MSC 2182
Bethesda, MD 20892-2182
http://nccam.nih.gov/health/whatiscam

**World Health Organization**
Avenue Appia 20
1211 Geneva 27
Switzerland
http://www.who.int/about/en/

*Good Health/Good Sense* Whatever path an individual chooses to attain a healthful, balanced life, s/he will find the information presented by Dr. Andrew Weil (2011) extremely sensible, thorough, and helpful in obtaining optimum physical and emotional health. Written in an engaging, relaxed style and backed by sound scientific evidence, *Spontaneous Happiness* offers a practical foundation for understanding emotional dis-ease and for seeking contentment, resilience, emotional balance, and comfort; the work also offers advice and guidance in developing spiritual dimensions of our lives. Dr Weil's work draws from both Eastern and Western psychological concepts and research and from mindfulness training as well as from nutritional science to weave a rich tapestry of strategies that support wellness. In the final chapters of this engaging work, Dr. Weil presents an eight-week program that results in better sleep, more energy, less stress, fewer illnesses, and a revitalized mental outlook.

In addition to *Spontaneous Happiness,* Dr. Weil is author of works on altered states of consciousness (*The Natural Mind: An Investigation of Drugs and the Higher Consciousness*), healthcare concerns of the elderly (*Healthy Aging*), healthcare reform (*Why Your Heath Matters*), and numerous other works on health and healing. Dr. Weil took part in the award-winning documentary *Escape Fire: The Fight to Rescue American Healthcare* which premiered in 2012 at the Sundance Film Festival and was released on DVD in 2013.

The Arizona Center for Integrative Medicine at the University of Arizona College of Medicine was founded by Dr. Weil with primary focus on education, clinical care, and research. In his deliberations for establishing the institution, Dr. Weil made significant distinctions between "integrative" and "alternative" medical practices. Any medicine or medical practice traditionally excluded from conventional practices may be seen as "alternative" — generally closer to natural remedies, cheaper, and less invasive than conventional therapies. Some may be scientifically validated; many are not. Likewise some conventional therapies are scientifically validated; some are not. When an alternative medical practice is applied in conjunction with a conventional one, the practice or medicine is referred to as "complementary".

Integrative medical practice, by contrast, is concerned with appropriate, scientifically validated therapies that facilitate the body's innate healing response and take into account the patient's body, mind, and spirit. Integrative medicine neither rejects nor accepts therapies uncritically, and it seeks natural, least invasive interventions when possible. Emphasis is on promoting good health and preventing illness as well as treating disease.

It is not surprising, then, that many principles and practices in **Ayurvedic ("life knowledge") medicine** are being incorporated into integrated healthcare practices because of its emphasis on *prevention* of disease and treatment of illness by way of maintaining *balance* in the body, mind, and consciousness. Considered by many practitioners to be the oldest healing science (practiced in India for over 5000 years), Ayurveda is a holistic approach to health that emphasizes the role of consciousness in maintaining good health and highlights the expression of positive emotions to attune one's life with the natural rhythms of the body. It is interesting to note the overall cancer incidence in the United States, in spite of billions of dollars spent on research each year, has not changed significantly in the last half-century. Cancers of the prostate, breast, lung, and colon, although most common in the Western world, are least common in the Eastern world.

The Integrative Medicine Center at the University of Maryland (University, 2013) explains that Ayurveda holds the belief that just as everyone has a unique fingerprint, each person has a distinct pattern of energy. The center offers this brief explanation of three basic energy types (doshas*):*

**Vata** — Energy that controls bodily functions associated with motion, including blood circulation, breathing, blinking, and heartbeat. When vata energy is balanced, there is creativity and vitality. Out of balance, vata produces fear and anxiety.

**Pitta** — Energy that controls the body's metabolic systems, including digestion, absorption, nutrition, and temperature. In balance, pitta leads to contentment and intelligence. Out of balance, pitta can cause ulcers and arouse anger.

**Kapha** — Energy that controls growth in the body. It supplies water to all body parts, moisturizes the skin, and maintains the immune system. In balance, kapha is expressed as love and forgiveness. Out of balance, kapha leads to insecurity and envy.

The underlying concept of Ayurvedic medical practice is that the mind and body are one as are the interactive and interdependent mental and physical realities. Balance is a critical issue in the three energy types (which correspond to Wind, Fire, and Earth), and treatment almost always includes recommendations for changes in lifestyle, especially diet. Many Ayurvedic practitioners recommend a vegetarian diet that can lower blood pressure and cholesterol and speed recovery from illness. Much of the medicine itself is plant-based but may contain some animal products. Some recent controversies have arisen about the quality of herbal supplements used in Ayurvedic practice, and the World Health Organization has taken on the task of monitoring usage and proposing worldwide quality standards. Some herbal supplements may also interact with conventional prescriptions and need to be monitored by a qualified practitioner. A list of Ayurvedic centers and qualified practitioners in the United States is available from:

---

**The National Institute of Ayurvedic Medicine (NIAM):**
www.panchakarma.com/the-national-institute-of-ayurvedic-medicine,-new-york,-usa-p-342.html.

Other sources of information include:
**California Association of Ayurvedic Medicine** --
www.ayurveda-caam.org
**Ayurvedic Institute** -- www.ayurveda.com

---

One of the many benefits that has emerged from the recent growth of Integrative Medicine in Western healthcare is a willingness of traditional practitioners and researchers to consider or reconsider the value of some common and not-so-common healthcare practices. Family practitioners and nutritionists are speaking to one another, as are chiropractors and surgeons, acupuncturists and neurologists. Curiosity, funding, new technologies, and dedicated research over time will help unravel some of the knots in our understanding of what works and why so that patients can make healthcare decisions with greater awareness and trust.

One such undertaking lies in a field of inquiry called *"Energetics"* which explores mechanisms by which mind and body processes influence the body's healing and performance potential. Research in the field draws on an extraordinary range of sources — from physiology and biophysics to inquiry into "spontaneous healing," aging, cutting-edge athletic and artistic performance, the martial arts, acupuncture, and numerous contemplative and spiritual practices. By providing new insights and theoretical models, this research field seeks ways to apply new information practically and clinically in such therapies as myofascial release, emotional freedom techniques, Reiki healing, Yoga, meditation, reconnective healing, and various kinesthetic therapies.

A leading spokesman for energetics medicine is Dr. James L. Oschman, author of numerous research works published in the *Journal of Bodywork and Movement Therapies* and several books that should acquaint readers with the theoretical basis for exploring the physiology and biophysics of energy medicines. Dr. Oschman is founder and president of Nature's Own Research Association located in Dover, New Hampshire, and is a member of the Scientific Advisory Board for the National Foundation for Alternative Medicine in Washington, DC, which is researching electromagnetic devices for treating cancer. His books include *Energy Medicine: The Scientific Basis (2004)* and *Energy Medicine in Therapeutics and Human Performance. (2004)*. Also interesting in this field are works by David F. Mayor and Marc S. Micozzi, *Energy Medicine East and West: A Natural History of Qi* (2011) and by Carolyn McMakin, *Frequency Specific Microcurrent in Pain Management* (2011).

Police officers seldom benefit from ignoring information, even untested information gleaned from experience in the field. Survival in high-stress situations does not preclude intuition or "street smarts, and many veteran officers, especially field operatives, have related that they have knowledge, and use, of energy interactions they have gained by non-scientific, experiential, and phenomenological testing. For readers who are reluctant to investigate emerging or alternative healthcare practices, it may be encouraging to keep in mind that what is "fringe" today may be leading-edge tomorrow because of new measuring technologies and investigators' dedication.

**Beyond Pain Management.** Another fruitful outgrowth of Integrative Medicine is new information on pain management accompanied by dramatic changes in the way we understand and treat pain. For example, research by Professor Fadel Zeidan and colleagues (Zeidan et al., 2011) sought to determine the brain mechanisms that support mediation of pain during mindfulness meditation while a wealth of other studies seek to understand how pain is perceived and processed, how it may alter the entire nervous system , and how it acts to alter thoughts and emotions. Stanford University's Systems Neuroscience and Pain Lab at the Stanford School of Medicine reports that over 100 million Americans suffer from debilitating chronic pain, and the goal of the pain lab is to translate research discoveries into effective therapies. The website http://snapldev.stanford.edu/news/ provides extensive information on recent and ongoing research.

It is not the intent of this work to offer testimonials for specific healing therapies; however, several contributors to this work have experienced remarkable "alternative" therapies. Aware of the many steps and controversies involved in integrating new information into mainstream practices, we offer some general information for readers' consideration.

*Myofascial Release Therapy* is a noninvasive form of soft-tissue manipulation used to treat impaired functioning of skeletal, arthroidial, and myofascial structures and associated lymphatic, neural, and vascular systems. The therapy addresses pain and restricted motion related to impaired functions and may be particularly effective with such conditions as sciatica, neck and shoulder restrictions, carpel tunnel, chronic fatigue syndrome, chronic back pain, fibromyalgia, temporomanibular joint disorders (TMJ), injuries, and reduced range-of-motion conditions that may not respond to more conventional approaches. The therapy is accomplished by relaxing contracted muscles, increasing lymphatic drainage, improving circulation, stimulating muscular stretch reflexes, and stimulating overlying fascia, which is the soft tissue element of connective tissue in the human body. The connective tissue provides support and protection for muscles and other body structures. The intent is to re-trigger the body's own healing functions which may have been suppressed; that is, the brain may have "shut down" a nerve reaction in order for the body to experience less pain at a given moment. The therapy essentially re-triggers the nervous system to take care of neglected areas, allowing the psychophysical body to heals itself by paying attention to its damages and by healing them with its own powers. A similar restorative process occurs during sleep. The REM cycle of sleep, in fact, is called the most restorative state of human existence.

Myofascial therapy recognizes that the body's soft tissue may become restricted as a result of overuse, trauma, infections, inactivity, or psychogenic disease, often resulting in pain, muscle tension, and diminished blood flow. Myofascial release therapy has also been tested as a recovery regimen after high-intensity exercise and associated heart rate and blood pressure conditions (Arroyo-Morales et al., 2008); Additionally, many chiropractic practitioners are currently merging myofascial therapy techniques into their treatments. Two of the most common forms of myofascial release therapy are the **John F. Barnes** and **Bowen Therapy.**

The New York Academy of Nutrition notes that it offers students access to more than 100 dietary theories. Unless the reader is endowed with an innate and powerful media-filtering system, s/he might wonder if 100 theories are adequate. There are special diets for athletes, special diets for specific athletic activities, special diets for specific diseases, diets for those who want to lose weight and for those who want to gain weight, vegan diets, high-protein meat and fat-based diets . . . . Many are thoughtful and effective; many are popular; many more are untested and may be nutritionally unsound.

The words "nutrition" and "diet" are not synonymous, nor are "controversy" and "condemnation." One way to check information overload at the door and to sort out fact from fiction may simply be to "read the label" and make individual efforts to understand agenda, bias, and subjectivity. The truth may be individual and not available in patented sizes and shapes, shrink-wrapped and ready for mass distribution. Critical thinking goes hand-in-hand with sound nutrition and sound healthcare decisions.

In this work, we look at two highly publicized diet therapies, one of which — **Gerson Therapy** — reads rather like a mystery novel. Before the midpoint of the 20th century, German physician Max Gerson developed a dietary therapy originally intended to treat migraine headaches and tuberculosis but soon promoted as a cure for cancer and a number of chronic, degenerative diseases. When poisoned by arsenic, Dr. Gerson applied his own therapy and survived the poisoning. Upon returning to his practice, Dr. Gerson found that his soon-to-be-published manuscript relating to the therapy was missing. He was murdered shortly after rewriting and publishing the text. The murder case was never solved, but among the suspects was, of course, an agency that would likely make fortunes from cancer therapies over the next 75 years. Dr. Gerson's daughter, Charlotte Gerson, subsequently founded the nonprofit Gerson Institute to provide education and training services aimed at treating chronic degenerative diseases. The institute is located in San Diego, California, and although the Gerson therapy is not practiced in the United States, it has followers and clinics in Mexico, Hungary, and Japan.

The rigorous therapy itself is considered a restorative approach to healthcare which targets the central issues of many diseases, namely nutritional deficiency and toxins. Fresh organic juices are used to dose the body with enzymes, nutrients, and minerals, and colonic treatments are prescribed to remove toxins from the body. Supplements are used to stimulate the metabolism, and excess animal proteins and fats are avoided, as are toxins and salt. In addition to the organic shake drinks, consumed many times throughout the day, there are solid foods that are combined with oxygenation techniques and consumed both raw and cooked. There are numerous classes, documentary films, videos, and books relating to the Gerson program. The institute office is located at 3844 Adams Avenue, San Diego, California. The mailing address is P.O. Box 161358, San Diego, CA, 92176, and the website is www.gerson.org/gerpress/

In contrast to the rigors and controversies of the Gerson diet, Dr. Dean Ornish maintains that lifestyle changes, including dietary considerations in particular, can dynamically and rapidly assist in attaining and sustaining better health. It may be that the simple *choices* a person makes are actually the "best medicine" one can "take." The relatively simple proactive program offered by the *Ornish Spectrum* focuses on four elements and may be undertaken at any level of engagement, depending on the wishes, interests, and time constraints of participants

**What you eat**

**How you respond to stress**

**How much activity you have**

**How much love and support you have**

*Source:* www.**ornishspectrum**.com

Dr. Ornish is affiliated with the non-profit organization Preventive Medicine Research Institute which collaborates with the University of California, San Francisco and other academic institutions to conduct research and develop sound nutrition and diet programs. Among his books are *Dr. Dean Ornish's Program for Reversing Heart Disease: The Only System Scientifically Proven to Reverse Heart Disease Without Drugs or Surgery* and *The Spectrum: A Scientifically Proven Program to Feel Better, Live Longer, Lose Weight, and Gain Health.* Dr. Ornish also participates in the Food Revolution Network (website: www. foodrevolution.org/blog/dr-ornish/) and is a frequent speaker for that organization on the subject or preventing disease and promoting health. Many other books on nutrition, diet, and lifestyle available through the Food Revolution Network, other websites, and bookstores are listed on the following page.

*The Engine 2 Diet: The Texas Firefighter's 28-Day Save-Your-Life Plan that Lowers Cholesterol and Burns Away the Pounds*
— Rip Esselstyn

*The Food Revolution: How Your Diet Can Help Save Your Life and Our World*

*Diet For A New America: How Your Food Choices Affect Your Health, Happiness, and the Future of Life on Earth*

*The Awakened Heart: Meditations on Finding Harmony in a Changing World*
— John Robbins

*The Kind Diet: A Simple Guide to Feeling Great, Losing Weight, and Saving the Planet* — Alicia Silverstone

*No More Bull!: The Mad Cowboy Targets America's Worst Enemy: Our Diet*
— Howard F. Lyman with Glen Merzer & Joanna Samorow-Merzer

*Skinny Bitch: A No-Nonsense, Tough-Love Guide for Savvy Girls Who Want to Stop Eating Crap and Start Looking Fabulous*
—Rory Freedman and Kim Barnouin

*Quantum Wellness: A Practical Guide to Health and Happiness*
—Kathy Freston

*Women Food and God: An Unexpected Path to Almost Everything*
— Geneen Roth

*A Course in Weight Loss: 21 Spiritual Lessons for Surrendering Your Weight Forever* —Marianne Williamson

*The Green Foodprint: Food Choices for Healthy People and a Healthy Planet*
— Linda Riebel

*Harvest for Hope: A Guide to Mindful Eating*
—Jane Goodall with Gary McAvoy and Gail Hudson

*Hope's Edge: The Next Diet for a Small Planet*
—Frances Moore Lappé and Anna Lappé

*The Hundred-Year Lie: How to Protect Yourself from the Chemicals That Are Destroying Your Health* — Randall Fitzgerald

*Eat Here: Reclaiming Homegrown Pleasures in a Global Supermarket*
—Brain Halweil

*The War on Bugs* — Will Allen

*Eaarth: Making a Life on a Tough New Planet* — Bill McKibben

*Super Immunity: The Essential Nutrition Guide for Boosting Your Body's Defenses to Live Longer, Stronger, and Disease Free*
— Joel Fuhrman

*Prevent and Reverse Heart Disease: The Revolutionary, Scientifically Proven, Nutrition-Based Cure* — Caldwell Esselstyn, M.D.

*The China Study: Startling Implications for Diet, Weight Loss and Long Term Health* — T. Collin Campbell, Ph.D.

*Food for Life: How the New Four Food Groups Can Save Your Life*
— Neal Barnard, M.D.

***The Power of Botanicals.*** "Take willow bark and see me in the morning" is not an unlikely prescription for medical treatment that predates written history. The bark of willow trees contains salicylic acid, the active metabolite of aspirin, and archeological evidence suggests that human beings have been using medicinal plants to treat disease and ailments for perhaps 60,000 years. Written records date back about 5,000 years to a Sumerian clay tablet that lists hundreds of medicinal plants; another early written record is the *Ebers Papyrus*, an Egyptian compendium of medical information that dates from around. 1550 BC and contains information on over 850 plant preparations. Readers may enjoy knowing that the Ebers Papyrus contains a prescription for *Cannabis sativa* (marijuana) applied topically for inflammation; it also recommends "half an onion and the froth of beer" as a "delightful remedy against death" (source and translation undetermined, but perhaps interesting to contemplate.)

The study of plants used as medicines — ethnobotany — has an absorbing and extremely rich history, but we should perhaps fast-forward to the 21st Century where controversy may be more common than compendia. According to the World Health Organization, the use herbal medicines is almost universal in non-industrialized societies and widely used in Ayurvedic, Chinese, and Tibetan herbal medicine; in addition, about 25 percent of modern drugs — aspirin, digitalis, quinine, and opium, for example — used in the United States have been derived from plants. Despite wide-spread usage and the fact that many herbal medicines can be grown from seed at very low cost, there are a number of controversies and concerns about methods of extraction, quality, safety, and efficacy. In addition, there are medical concerns about the interactions of herbs and pharmaceutical drugs, as some herbal remedies may interfere with or amplify the effects of prescription drugs.

The primary agency of the United States government responsible for biomedical and health-related research is the National Institutes of Health, and the Food and Drug Administration is responsible for overseeing herbal remedies, which are regulated as dietary supplements. Although manufacturers of products in this category are not required to prove the safety or effectiveness of products they produce, the FDA may withdraw a product from sale should it prove harmful. In the European Union herbal medicines are regulated under the European Directive on Traditional Herbal Medicinal Products. The World Health Organization works with member states to establish quality standards for herbal medicines.

Research in herbal medicines is frequently fueled by pharmaceutical companies interested in future drug development. Working in the Program for Collaborative Research in the Pharmaceutical Sciences, College of Pharmacy, University of Illinois-Chicago, for example, researchers D.S. Fabricant and N.R. Farnsworth

(2001) studied advantages and disadvantages of plants used in traditional medicine for drug discovery, reporting that they had identified 122 compounds obtained from 94 species of plants that are used globally as drugs. In 2009, the National Institutes of Health sponsored a consortium of researchers at Washington State University, the Donald Danforth Plant Science Center, the National Center for Genome Resources, Santa Fe, and the University of Illinois to study medicinal plant species and begin developing a medicinal plant transcriptomics database. Extensive evidence-based information for pharmacists and other healthcare professionals on recent research is available in the publication *Herbal Medicines* , *3rd edition* (Barnes, Phillipson, & Anderson, 2007) and in the updated 4th edition available in 2013 from the Pharmaceutical Press (London).

For the less academically inclined, there are numerous publications and a thoughtful, practical website maintained by the **American Herbalist Guild** (www.americanherbalist.com.). Nor are the whimsical and fanciful readers, magicians, and sorcerers among us to be overlooked. Two of the most engaging works are Scott Cunningham's *Magical Herbalism: The Secret Craft of the Wise* (Cunningham, 2001) and Ann Moira's works, which include *Green Witchcraft: Folk Magic, Fairy Lore, and Herb Craft* (Moira, 1999). And finally, for the insatiably curious reader, the "flower of life" — not an herb but a geometrical symbol — has a long history of influence in music, architecture, mathematics, and in spiritual quests. (See Melchizedek, 1999 and 2000, for an introduction to fractals and an adventure into subjects as varied as sacred geometry, the tree of life, the Fibonacci sequence, the golden ratio, solfeggio harmonics, and divine order. The message from these works may simply be that the more a person can conform to the natural flow and shape of life, the more likely it is that he/she will flow on in existence. A misshapen object will teeter and sink; a balanced object will flow.

Physicists and nurses, neuroscientists and musicians, sound engineers and psychologist, biologists and composers . . . are having a party. And it's all about music: Music and the brain, music and heart rate, music and speech/language, music as therapy, music and motor skills, music and perception, music and performance, music and education, music and healing. The first volume of *The Neurosciences and Music,* published by the New York Academy of Sciences in 2003, contained 70 research papers concerned with how the creation and perception of music related to brain activity and anatomy. The second volume, published in 2006, contained 56 papers concerned with perception and performance. Ninety research works graced Volume III (2009) which focused on disorders and plasticity, and the 2012 publication of Volume IV contained 47 research papers exploring learning and memory. By any standards, that's a lot of research in a nine-year span – and a lot of celebrating. New technologies in brain-imaging and other advanced research techniques provide greater and greater understanding of how music influences mood; how music may enhance intelligence, mental health, and the immune system; how music may enhance memory and performance on cognitive tests; how music therapy may lower cortisol levels and reduce stress, anxiety, and depression.

Dr. Daniel J. Levitin, cognitive neuroscientist at McGill University in Montreal, has made these statements about music and health:

> We've found compelling evidence that musical interventions can play a health care role in settings ranging from operating rooms to family clinics. But even more importantly, we were able to document the neurochemical mechanisms by which music has an effect in four domains: management of mood, stress, immunity and as an aid to social bonding. . . . I think the promise of music as medicine is that it's natural and it's cheap and it doesn't have the unwanted side effects that many pharmaceutical products do.

> Dr. Levitin is author of *This Is Your Brain on Music: The Science of Human Obsession (2006)* and *The World in Six Songs: How the Musical Brain Created Human Nature (2008)* and is director of the Laboratory for Music Cognition, Perception and Expertise at McGill University.

Each of us likely has favorite songs or type of music; we may enjoy particular eras or niches in musical style. Indeed, access to music appears to be an unquestioned aspect of life, and for some theorists, it is the very stuff of our existence, with sound vibrations in various constructs being the building blocks of reality (Erneling & Johnson, 2004; Gell-Mann, 2010; and Vaillant, 2003) . History is resplendent with physicists and philosophers alike who come to the conclusion that music is a tuning frequency vibration with the power to heal, to communicate joy and wellness, and to share knowledge and wisdom. Not the least of these was Dr. Albert Einstein (physicist and musician) who many times explained that his most important thoughts developed not with symbols, but initially with images, music, and intuition. He coined the term "musicality" when speaking about Niels Bohr's work on the structure of the atom. Einstein said that Bohr's work was "the highest form of *musicality* in the realm of thought" (Calaprice, 2000).

Some research suggests that it doesn't have to be "good" music that promotes healing, just music that appeals to the individual – for whatever reasons. The Solfeggio frequency, for example, and the basic neuro-frequencies of both the earth and ourselves, are believed to have the power to create positive shifts in our well-being. Some things just sing, and we can look to science and theory, music and the arts, to guide us into a world of greater harmony if only we lend an ear.

During Academy training, police officers are introduced to multicultural diversity, multicultural awareness, and cultural competency training; they learn the pitfalls of racial profiling, and they are encouraged to examine their own belief systems as a first step in embracing racial and cultural diversity, appreciation, and acceptance. Our training, however, seems to draw an invisible line at consideration of religious beliefs or spiritual paths or affinities, as if that "other realm" were either irrelevant or dangerous territory. In the US Army Comprehensive Fitness Program, spirituality is one of five dimensions (physical, emotional, social, family, and spiritual) considered important in strengthening soldiers' resilience and enhancing performance, although there have been numerous criticisms that the spiritual element is not well integrated into a holistic fitness program.

Frequently for individuals, it isn't until the onset of trauma or debilitating disease that the mind allows itself to venture into unexplored territory. The authors of this work offer here some brief information about spiritual paths that may be useful to the reader who is seeking healing and enhanced well-being. This information is by no means a recruiting memo, but rather an invitation to consider well-being in a holistic fashion in which concepts of peace, justice, learning, and service hold hands with practical regimens for healthful diets, routine exercise, and sound restorative sleep. Our intent is not to promote a particular concept or even to celebrate diversity and difference, but rather to suggest healing paths that acknowledge the strengths and the unity of all humankind. By making efforts to understand the pitfalls of habituated thinking and emotive turbulence, a reader is inevitably reminded of how inquiry into learning and into spirituality has powerful ramifications for well-being.

In the *Bahá'í Faith*, for example – with an estimated five to six million members in more than 200 countries and territories — humanity is seen to be in a process of collective evolution in which the current need is the establishment of global peace, justice, and unity. Religious history is seen to have progressed over time through divine messengers suited to the capacities of the people and the requirements of the time. These messengers have included Moses, Buddha, Jesus, Muhammad, and others; for Baha'is, the most recent messengers are the Báb and Bahá'u'lláh. Essential elements in the teachings and goals of the faith include a relentless search for truth, unimpaired by superstition, bigotry, or prejudice; harmony between religion and science; equality of men and women; compulsory education and pursuit of learning ; ennobling of work in the service of others; the exaltation of justice in human society, and the establishment of a permanent and universal peace.

If we are concerned with the unity of all humankind, it is not surprising that some of these elements have a familiar ring in the swearing-in statement from the International Association of Chiefs of police regarding peace officers' responsibilities:

> *My fundamental duty is to serve mankind; safeguard lives and property; protect the innocent against deception, the weak against oppression or intimidation, and the peaceful against violence or disorder, and respect the Constitutional rights of all to liberty, equality, and justice.*

Police officers may frequently see themselves as warriors, sometimes wounded warriors, rather than as guardians and keepers of the peace so it may be both fruitful and pleasing to consider the concept of "spiritual warriors" as presented by don Miguel Ruiz in his Toltec Wisdom books, including *The Four Agreements: A Practical Guide to Personal Wisdom* (Ruiz, 1997) and *Beyond Fear: A Toltec Guide to Freedom and Joy: The Teachings of don Miguel Ruiz*, as recorded by Mary Carroll Nelson (Nelson & Ruiz, 1997). The four agreements are 1) Be impeccable with your word; 2) Don't take anything personally; 3) Don't make assumptions; and 4) Always do your best.

Don Miguel Ruiz sees the spiritual warrior as someone who has decided to adopt the agreements and to challenge the fear-based beliefs in his/her mind and to address limiting belief systems in the individual's social environment. Thus, the warrior's challenge is not to confront an external enemy, but rather to engage in an internal transformation.

In Toltec practice, the transformation process is aided by attention to messages from an individual's dream state and by ceremonies engaging the energies of a group. The purpose of the practice (Mitote) is to increase awareness of how throughout the day we shift from conscious to subconscious awareness and how we may learn to take more control in both the dream and the waking states in order to move from reactive modes of behavior to proactive modes. The individual has opportunities to understand self-imposed limitation — mental and emotional responses based on habituated or patterned reactions — and to consider the personal power of choice and conscious intention to alter our situations in life.

The evolution of social consciousness may be one of the most studied concepts in modern thought, but one need not be an historian nor a scholar in any discipline to find wisdom and inspiration in the eloquent words of Lao Tzu, dating from the sixth century, BC. Verse 8 of the *Tao Te Ching* states:

The highest good is like water,
nourishing life effortlessly,
flowing without prejudice
to the lowliest places.
It springs from all
who nourish their community
with a benevolent heart as deep as an abyss,
who are incapable of lies and injustices,
who are rooted in the earth,
and whose natural rhythms of action
play midwife to the highest good
of each pregnant moment.

This verse is reprinted from a new translation, with commentary, of *Tao Te Ching*, a stunning work by Ralph Alan Dale with memorable photographs by John Cleare (Dale, 2005, p. 17). The work also includes a chart of the development of society and consciousness with the yin epoch characterized as tribal societies, the yang epoch characterized as coercive civilizations. The future is characterized as an expression of planetary holism—what Lao Tzu saw as "the Great Integrity." The chart shows the evolution of law, for example, as moving from taboos to preserve the integrity of tribes, through laws to preserve property rights, to a future of universal ethics to preserve the Great Integrity. Social relations are shown as moving from the small harmony of tribal communes, through the great fragmentation of competition and aggression, to a future of the great harmony in a planetary community.

We close this section with some recent comments by His Holiness the Fourteenth Dalai Lama:

*I believe that each individual should embark upon a spiritual path that is best suited to his or her mental disposition, natural inclination, temperament, belief, family, and cultural background.*
from *The Art of Happiness: A Handbook for Living*
(Gyatso & Cutler,1998).

*Much of human suffering stems from destructive emotions, as hatred breeds violence and craving fuels addiction.*
from *Destructive Emotions: A Scientific Dialogue with the Dalai Lama* (Goleman & Gyatso, 2003), narrated by Professor Daniel Goleman, author of *Emotional Intelligence*, co-founder of the Collaborative for Academic, Social, and Emotional Learning at Yale University's Child Studies Center, and a board member of the Mind Life Institute.

Following is a list of other works by the Dalai Lama and some of his collaborative works with noted scholars.

*Becoming Enlightened*
> Jeffrey Hopkins, Narrator, Translator
> Atria/Simon &Schuster

*Beyond Religion: Ethics for a Whole World*
> With contributions from Alexander Norman
> Houghton Mifflin Harcourt Publishing

*Consciousness at the Crossroads: Conversations with the Dalai Lama on Brain Science and Buddhism*
> Zara Houshmand, B. Alan Wallace, and Robert B. Livingston, Editors; Snow Lion Publications

*The Dalai Lama's Book of Wisdom:* Harper

*Freedom in Exile: The Autobiography of the Dalai Lama:*     Harper

*Gentle Bridges: Conversations with the Dalai Lama on the Sciences of Mind.*
> Jeremy W. Hayward and Francisco J. Varela.
> Shambhala Publications

*Healing Anger: The Power Of Patience From A Buddhist Perspective*
> Thupten Jinpa, Translator; Snow Lion Publications

*Healing Emotions: Conversations with the Dalai Lama on Mindfulness, Emotions, and Health*
> Daniel Goleman; Shambhala Publications

*How to Practice: The Way to a Meaningful Life*
> Jeffrey Hopkins, Editor and Translator
> Simon and Schuster

*How to See Yourself As You Really Are*
> Jeffrey Hopkins, Narrator, Translator; Atria Books

*In My Own Words: An Introduction to My Teachings and Philosophy*
> Rajiv Mehrotra, Translator; Hay House Publishing

*Mind and Life: Discussions with the Dalai Lama on the Nature of Reality (Columbia Series in Science and Religion)*
> Pier Luigi Luisi. Zara Houshmand, Editor
> Columbia University Press

*My Land and My People: The Original Autobiography of His Holiness the Dalai Lama of Tibet*
> Warner Books

*The New Physics and Cosmology: Dialogues with the Dalai Lama*
> Arthur Zajonc and Zara Houshmand, Editors,
> Oxford University Press

*An Open Heart: Practicing Compassion in Everyday Life*
> Nicolas Vreeland, Contributor
> Little, Brown and Company

*Sleeping, Dreaming, and Dying: An Exploration of Consciousness with the Dalai Lama*
> Francisco J. Varela, Editor
> Wisdom Publications

*Stages of Meditation*
> Geshe Lobsang Jordhen, Losang Choephel Ganchenpa, and
> Jeremy Russell, Translators
> Snow Lion Publications

*Toward a True Kinship of Faiths: How the World's Religions Can Come Together*
> Doubleday

*The Universe in a Single Atom: The Convergence of Science and Spirituality*
> Morgan Road Books/Random House

*Visions of Compassion: Western Scientists and Tibetan Buddhists Examine Human Nature*
> Richard J. Davidson and Anne Harrington, Editors
> Oxford University Press

# The Global Coherence Initiative

Research conducted by contributors to this work has taken us on many paths, some perhaps discouraging, others energizing and illuminated by hope, compassion, empathy, and joy. In these final pages, we offer a look at some of the amazing work being done to advance our understanding of stress-related illness and to bolster our opportunities for individual, community, and global well- being.

Dr. Rollin McCraty, Research Director for the Institute of HeartMath, has graciously given us permission to relate and discuss some of on-going research work at the Institute as reported in an article *The Global Coherence Initiative: Creating a Coherent Planetary Standing Wave* (McCraty, Deyhle, & Childre, 2012).Working with geologist and marine geochemist Annette Deyhle and with Institute of HeartMath founder Doc Childre, McCraty presented evidence for the existence of a global information field that connects all living systems and consciousness. The researchers stated:

> The convergence of several independent lines of evidence provides strong support for the existence of a global information field that connects all living systems and consciousness. Every cell in our bodies is bathed in an external and internal environment of fluctuating invisible magnetic forces that can affect virtually every cell and circuit in biological systems. Therefore, it should not be surprising that numerous physiological rhythms in humans and global collective behaviors are not only synchronized with solar and geomagnetic activity, but disruptions in these fields can create adverse effects on human health and behavior (p. 64 ).

To understand and fully appreciate this astonishing statement, let's take a look at some of the work and the discoveries that lead to this conclusion and consider the implications for collaboratively addressing some of society's significant social, environmental, and economic problems while enhancing the well-being of individuals, families, workplaces, and communities.

Early in his career, Russian scientist Alexander Tchijevsky (1897 – 1964) noted that peak sunspot events coincided with the most severe World War I battles. He subsequently studied global human history between the years 1749 and 1926 and constructed an index of important political and social events such as the start of wars, social revolution, etc. in 72 countries. He then created a chart of solar cycles over the same time period. The two charts — solar cycles and "mass human activity"— were nearly identical, with 80 percent of the most significant events occurring during solar maximum, the highest period of geomagnetic activity. The charts are reproduced in the article *The Global Coherence Initiative: Creating a Coherent Planetary Standing Wave* (McCraty, Deyhle, & Childre, 2012, page 68, website: www.gahmj.com).

Subsequent studies revealed evidence that criminal activity accelerates during periods of increased solar activity; that a large shift occurred in the earth's geomagnetic field at the same time as the 9/11 terrorist attack on the World Trade Center; that the Iraq invasion of Kuwait took place during solar cycle peaks; and that social unrest in the Middle East synchronized with the solar cycle that began in 2011 and that will reach its peak in 2013-2014.

Scientific research has established that resonating geomagnetic frequencies occur in the earth-ionosphere resonant cavity and that these frequencies directly overlap with those of the human brain and cardio vascular system. The nature and extent of geomagnetic influences on the human brain, consciousness, behavior, and interactions, and the collective emotional responses reflected in the earth's ionosphere and geomagnetic field are the subjects of research currently being conducted by the Institute of HeartMath and the Global Coherence Initiative, a nonprofit research and education organization that seeks science-based information that may facilitate a shift in human consciousness — a shift away from instability toward intentional balance and fruitful cooperative efforts on a global scale.

The hypotheses that guide the Global Coherence Initiative/HeartMath research are listed here.(Readers are encouraged to see page 35 of this work for a discussion of the term "coherence".)

---

- That all living systems are interconnected at an energetic level and communicate via biological fields, including nonlocal fields, when certain conditions are met;
- That humans are affected by planetary energetic fields, and conversely, the earth's energetic systems are influenced by and act as a carrier wave for collective human emotions and consciousness (positively and negatively);
- That large numbers of people intentionally generating heart-coherent positive emotional states of care, compassion, love, and appreciation will generate a coherent standing wave that can help offset present and future planetary-wide standing waves of stress, fear, discord, and incoherence;
- That human emotions and consciousness interact with and encode information in planetary energetic fields, including the geomagnetic field, thereby communicating information between people at a subconscious level, which in effect, links all living systems and gives rise to a form of collective consciousness.

Source: *The Global Coherence Initiative: Creating a Coherent Planetary Standing Wave* (McCraty, Deyhle, & Childre, 2012) website: www.gahmj.com.

---

The current focus of the initiative is the continuing construction of a global coherence monitoring system that measures and explores fluctuations and resonances in the earth's magnetic field and in the earth-ionosphere resonant cavity in order to 1) investigate how the earth's fields affect human mental and emotional processes, health outcomes, and collective human behavior; 2) explore how collective human emotional states and intentions are reflected in the earth's electromagnetic and energetic fields; 3) determine if changes in those fields occur prior to natural disturbances such as earthquakes, volcanic eruptions, storms, and human-made events such as social upheaval, unrest, and terrorist attacks, and 4) monitor global events to determine where collective heart-coherent prayers, meditations, and intentions can be fruitfully directed.

To carry out this research, scientists are installing a global network of ultrasensitive magnetic field detectors to measure magnetic resonances in the earth/ionosphere cavity, resonances that are generated by the vibrations of the earth's geomagnetic field lines, and ultra-low frequencies that occur in the earth's magnetic field. There already exist networks that measure the strength of earth magnetic field and geomagnetic disturbances, but until recently there has not been a global network of detectors that measure the various and varying signals that occur in the same range as human physiological frequencies. The new detectors are increasing understanding of how earth's fields affect us and is enhancing our understanding of the interconnections between solar and other external forces on the planetary field environment. Data acquired by the global monitors is stamped with time and global-positioning data, transmitted to a common server, and freely made available to other research groups in keeping with the a primary goal of the Global Coherence Initiative: To facilitate a growing awareness of humanity's interdependence with the earth and with each other. The researchers concluded:

> . . . even if we are not able to prove the encoding of human intention in the global fields in the next few years, we can facilitate a deeper understanding of the mechanisms by which human health and behaviors are modulated by the earth's fields and further clarify which aspects of the field environment mediate the varied and specific effects. More important is Global Coherence Initiative's primary goal, which is to motivate more people to work together in a more coherent and collaborative manner to increase harmony in the collective consciousness to alleviate social conflicts and to improve the environmental impact we have on the planet and assist in planetary evolution.
>
> **Source:** *The Global Coherence Initiative: Creating a Coherent Planetary Standing Wave* (McCraty, Deyhle, & Childre, 2012), p 76. website: www.gahmj.com.

Jack Canfield, co-creator of the *Chicken Soup for the Soul*® book series and founder of the Transformational Leadership Council (website: http://www.transformationalleadershipcouncil.com/) made this statement about the Initiative:

*"The Global Coherence Initiative is perhaps the greatest experiment
in the history of the world."*

---

**Global Coherence Initiative**
14700 West Park Ave.,
Boulder Creek, California 95006
http://www.glcoherence.org/

Among the many resources available at the website are a site map of the monitoring system, webinars, audio, video, and PDF downloads as well as articles and scientific research papers.

---

Selected references cited in the article on *The Global Coherence Initiative: Creating a Coherent Planetary Standing Wave* are listed here for readers who may enjoy the science behind the science of the Global Coherence Initiative.

1971. *Physical factors of the historical process.*
   A.L.Tchijevsky (V.P.de Smitt, translator)
1981. *Environmental power-frequency magnetic fields and suicide.*
   F.S. Perry, M. Reichmanis, A.A. Marino, & R.O. Becker
1987. *Chronobiology and psychiatric disorders.* A. Halaris
1987. *Geopsychology and geopsychopathology: Mental processes and disorders associated with geochemical and geophysical factors.* M.A. Persinger
1988. *Alleviating political violence through enhancing coherence in collective consciousness: Impact assessment analysis of the Lebanon war [dissertation].* J.L. Davies
1989. *Network structure from relational data: measurement and inference in four operational models.* R.T. Bradley & N. C. Roberts
1991. *Analysis of variance of REG experiments: Operator intention, secondary parameters, database structure.*
   R.D .Nelson, Y.H. Dobyns, B.J .Dunne, & R.G. Jahn
1993. *The undivided universe: An ontological interpretation of quantum theory.*
   D. Bohm & B.J. Hiley
1994. *Geomagnetic storms: association with incidence of depression as measured by hospital admission.* R.W. Kay
1995. *The interconnected universe: Conceptual foundations of transdisciplinary unified theory.* E. Laszlo
1995. *On the possibility of directly accessing every human brain by electromagnetic induction of the fundamental algorithms.* M.A. Persinger

1995. *Sudden unexpected death in epileptics following sudden, intense, increases in geomagnetic activity: Prevalence of effect and potential mechanisms.* M.A. Persinger & C. Psych

1996. *Cardiac coherence: A new, noninvasive measure of autonomic nervous system order.* W.A. Tiller, R. McCraty, & M. Atkinson

1997. *The conscious universe: The scientific truth of psychic phenomena.* D. Radin

1998. *Cosmophysical correlations of creative activity in cultural history.* S. Ertel

1998. *Effect of variations of the geomagnetic field and solar activity on human physiological indicators.* V.N. Doronin, V.A. Parfentěv, S.Z. ,Tleulin, et al.

1999. *Chronomes, time structures, for chronobioengineering for "a full life."* G. Cornelissen, et al.

1999. *Effects of group practice of the transcendental meditation program on preventing violent crime in Washington, D.C.: Results of the National Demonstration Project.* J.S. Hagelin et al.

2000. *Cross-spectrally coherent ~10.5- and 21-year biological and physical cycles, magnetic storms and myocardial infarctions.* F. Halberg, G. Cornelissen, K. Otsuka

2000. *Prayer: An ancient healing practice becomes new again.* A. Ameling

2002. *The energetic heart: Bioelectromagnetic interactions within and between people.* R. McCraty

2002. *Mass emotions apparently affect nominally random quantum processes: Interplanetary magnetic field polarity found critical, but how is causal path?* H.W. Wendt

2003. *The effect of geomagnetic storms on suicide.* C. Gordon & M. Berk

2004. *Electrophysiological evidence of intuition: Part 1. The surprising role of the heart.* R. McCraty, M. Atkinson, & R.T. Bradley

2004. *Electrophysiological evidence of intuition: Part 2. A system-wide process?* M. Atkinson. & R.T. Bradley

2004. *The grateful heart: The psychophysiology of appreciation.* R. McCraty & D. Childre

2005. *The rainbow and the worm: The physics of organisms.* M.W. Ho

2006. *The contingency of parameters of human encephalograms and Schumann resonance electromagnetic fields revealed in monitoring studies.* S.V. Pobachenko, A.G. Kolesnik, A.S.Borodin, & V.V. Kalyuzhin

2006. *Tchijevsky's disclosure: How the solar cycles modulate the history.* S.V. Smelyakov

2007. *The power of the collective.* J. Hagelin

2007. *Solar activity, revolutions and cultural prime in the history of mankind.* M. Mikulecky

2008. *The GCP event experiment: Design, analytical methods, results.* P. Bancel & R. Nelson

2008. *On the possible representation of the electromagnetic equivalents of all human memory within the earth's magnetic field: Implications of theoretical biology.* M. Persinger

2008. *Quantum shift in the global brain: How the new scientific reality can change us and our world.* E. Laszlo

2009. *The coherent heart: Heart-brain interactions, psychophysiological coherence, and the emergence of system-wide order.* R. McCraty, M. Atkinson, D. Tomasino, & R.T. Bradley

2009. *The end of materialism: How evidence of the paranormal is bringing science and spirit together.* C. Tart

2009. *Heliogeophysical factors as possible triggers of suicide terroristic acts.* P. Grigoryev, V. Rozanov, A. Vaiserman, & B. Vladimirskiy

2009. *New hope for correctional officers: An innovative program for reducing stress and health risks.* R. McCraty, M. Atkinson, L. Lipsenthal, & L. Arguelles

2010. *Cardiac coherence and PTSD in combat veterans.* J.P. Ginsberg, M.E. Berry, & D.A. Powell

2010. *Coherence: Bridging personal, social and global health.* R. McCraty & D. Childre

2010. *Coherence training improves cognitive functions and behavior in children with attention-deficit hyperactivity disorder: Cognitive functions and behavioral changes.* A. Lloyd, D. Brett, & K. Wesnes

2010. *Emotion self-regulation, psychophysiological coherence, and test anxiety: Results from an experiment using electrophysiological measures.* R.T. Bradley, R. McCraty, M. Atkinson, D. Tomasino, A. Daugherty, & L. Arguelles

2010. *The global coherence initiative: Measuring human-earth energetic interactions.* R.. McCraty

2010. *Nonlocality, intention, and observer effects in healing studies: Laying a foundation for the future.* S.A .Schwartz & L. Dossey

2010. *Prayer and spiritual practices for health reasons among American adults: The role of race and ethnicity.* F. Gillum & D.M. Griffith

2010. *Scientific evidence for the existence of a true noosphere: Foundation for a noo-constitution.* R.. Nelson.

2011. *Detecting mass consciousness: Effects of globally shared attention and emotion.* R. Nelson

2011. *Non-local intuition in entrepreneurs and non-entrepreneurs: Results of two experiments using electrophysiological measures.* R.T. Bradley, M. Gillin, R. McCraty, & M. Atkinson

2011. *Non-verbal communication of compassion: Measuring psychophysiologic effects.* K.J. Kemper & H.A. Shaltout

2011. *Time structures (chronomes) of the blood circulation, populations' health, human affairs and space weather.* F. Halberg, et al.

2012. *Achieving collective coherence: Group effects on heart rate variability, coherence and heart rhythm synchronization.* S.M. Morris

# Becoming a World-Class Performer:
## A Guide for Achieving Performance Excellence
J. E. Ruesch

Information about training for performance excellence can provide guidelines for police officers who seek to overcome stress-related afflictions and wish to develop a regimen to restore and promote good health. They will recognize the relevance of mind-body congruence and the healthful benefits of developing self-awareness, resilience, and sense of purpose.

Retired U.S. Army General Peter J. Schoomaker once said: "Peak performance is not a destination; it is a constant in life. We need to get good at it by applying these principles to the whole organization as a culture. . . . This needs to be part of our everyday lives." In a subsequent interview, General Schoomaker stated that he was referring to an individual commitment to adopt a *relentless pursuit of excellence* in all that one does. Performance excellence is the result of individuals' abilities to create a positive state of mind and develop the necessary skills for overcoming the challenges that lie before them. Excellence is not perfection. In fact, compulsively pursuing perfection often makes people afraid of making mistakes, potentially leading to performance paralysis and inaction. High performers learn to face their fears and shortcomings and to work through them. They are masters, not victims, of life's situations. They control the quality of their lives in the following ways:

> - Personal integrity and high ethical standards.
> - Character, moral concern, and spiritual values.
> - Desire to make a positive contribution to the world.
> - Inner strength, courage, and endurance.
> - A true sense of humility and concern for others.
> - Maturity and the willingness to accept responsibility for one's actions.
> - A calm purposefulness and vision with a passion for excellence.
> - A positive attitude, respect for others, and a love of life.
> - Self-discipline and the ability to sustain focus and concentration.
> - Desire to succeed, set and achieve new goals, and challenge oneself.
> - Ability to creatively solve problems and apply critical thinking to make decisions.
> - Ability to influence and bond with others in a team.
> - A good sense of humor and the ability to laugh at oneself.

Even the most detailed of performance plans entirely depend on individuals' ability to overcome obstacles and thrive in an atmosphere of constantly changing adverse variables that stand between them and their desired performance outcome. This is especially true for collective performances. When engaging in a demanding performance situation, it is essential to possess the ability to overcome obstacles in order to attain superior outcomes. A relentless pursuit of performance excellence facilitates the development of a personality structure that provides the capacity for "**mental toughness**" during times of adversity, hardship, or under unfavorable conditions without deviation from an established level of performance. Mental toughness describes a collection of attributes that allow a person to persevere through difficult situations and emerge without losing confidence.

A person's ability to be mentally tough depends largely on how well s/he has anticipated and prepared for adversity in advance. Individuals who are properly prepared for a task tend to embrace adverse situations. They view stressful circumstances in perspective and choose to interpret them in a less threatening manner. As a consequence of these optimistic appraisals, the impact of the stressful events is reduced and is less likely to negatively affect the health of the individual. In contrast, less prepared individuals tend to demonstrate avoidance of adverse situations. Research on self-reported stressors, real-life stressful experiences, and laboratory-induced stress supports this claim. Nevertheless, no matter how hard people prepare, they will inevitably face demands on their mind and body that take them beyond their ability to perform at their potential, and they may deviate from pre-established performance levels. Tough, demanding training pushes an individual to this point frequently in the pursuit of continuous growth.

**Resilience** reflects the ability of individuals to maintain relatively stable mental, emotional, or physical function throughout the course of an event. Essentially, it is the ability to prepare for, recover from, and adapt in the presence of adversity. Many people associate resilience as the ability to bounce back after a fall in performance levels; however, resilience has just as much to do with sustaining a performance level as it does with returning to it. It is the power or ability one has to sustain or return to an original or pre-established state, performance level, or position after deviating as a result of confronting adversity, hardship, or unfavorable conditions that placed demands on the mind, body, or spirit. Enduring hardship and sustaining high performance levels are critical components for building **resilience capacity**.

There are different levels of resiliency that are extremely relevant to a person's overall health and success in performances. The ability to recover mentally, physically, and emotionally following a demanding performance is essential to growth. The ability to quickly "bounce back" after a setback in the course of a performance situation is essential for sustainability at a high functioning level during execution of a task.

Resilience is sometimes thought of as a psychological process that facilitates optimum functioning in response to adversity in life; however, resilience is much more than that. A broader definition suggests that resilience may be seen as the mind and body's ability to adapt in the face of adversity and *thrive* in an atmosphere of competing demands. It is clear that some people are much better equipped to adapt in an environment of changing demands than others are. Achieving and sustaining the highest possible level of performance in a tough and demanding situation require one to be agile enough to adapt quickly and to be mentally prepared to meet adversity head on with the will to do what it takes to achieve greatness in a performance. Reaching and sustaining one's true performance potential and the ability to control performance outcomes require a higher than normal level of intimacy with **performance agility** — the ability to rapidly respond to change by adapting from an original, stable performance disposition to a new one that addresses a change in demand and enables one to return to a previous level of performance.

Researchers suggest that resilience has three components: resilient qualities, the resiliency process, and innate resilience. Resilient qualities measure the psychosocial qualities of resilient individuals. The resiliency process describes how the individual adapts to adversity, and innate resilience consists of the identification of motivational factors that may influence the individual's response. **Self-regulated resilience** has four prerequisites that directly contribute to the capacity a person possesses for performance agility:

> ➤ Risk or predisposition to bio-psychosocial or environmental conditions.
> ➤ Exposure to a high-magnitude distractions.
> ➤ Response to detractors of attention and other forms of adversity.
> ➤ Return to pre-established baseline of performance, functioning, and impedance levels..

## Performing at One's Potential

Performance excellence is the result of one's ability to create a positive state of mind and develop skills for overcoming challenges and internalizing the lessons one learns along the way. Setting high standards and applying oneself with attentiveness and determination leads to becoming a self-regulated high-level performer. Excellence in performance is not about achieving perfection. High-level performers learn to face adversity and work through it. It is critical to identify with detailed aspects of one's performance, make the necessary adjustments for increasing performance, and remember those adjustments in order to benefit from the learning. Whether in a college classroom, in a demanding business environment, or engaged in spatial conditioning on a practice field in the National Football League, learning is the key to growth reflected in an increase in resilience capacity.

World-class performers are no more nor less vulnerable to energy drain or distractions than any other person is. They have simply learned to overcome obstacles that interfere with superior performance through personalized training. The first step in putting together a strong training strategy is to isolate the cause of a distraction as it relates to a particular task or situation. Reaching and sustaining one's performance potential requires the successful navigation across tough and demanding situations full of unpredictable distractions. Every day there are unpredictable things that capture one's focus. When people choose to focus on distractions that are predictable, they can then make a plan to address and overcome the adversity.

The ability to attend in the present and stay focused on a task is referred to as "**mental agility**" and is pivotal to success in animated, fast-paced environments when adversity is at its highest. In competitive situations, as well as in everyday life, there are times when a person can feel somewhat overwhelmed by the complexity of a situation or task. Stress, operational tempo, unclear objectives, and lack of experience are all contributors and/or the results of ineffective attention control.

Perhaps the greatest factor in determining if individuals are going to reach performance excellence is their **motivation** — desire and energy directed toward achievement of a goal. In other words, a person without goals is not motivated. Contrary to what many believe, it is not human nature to excel at a task; it is more common for a person to provide only the amount of energy and focus needed for a perceived minimal acceptable effort. People need a reason to excel that is either for themselves or because of some outside influence that drives them. Successful leaders, managers, and coaches strive to provide their teams with detailed direction that instills a sense of purpose at a level that each team member considers personally valuable and that boosts individual productivity.

## Sharpening Focus and Concentration

Raising one's level of performance and sustaining it for long periods requires a degree of competency in these six areas:

> ➤ Effective Thinking
> ➤ Confidence
> ➤ Goal Setting
> ➤ Energy Management
> ➤ Mental Rehearsal
> ➤ Controlling attention

None of these domains is dominant over another, as each is interdependent; however, the ability to attend stands out as the control mechanism that orchestrates the success or failure of an individual's Personal Performance Plan (P3). Essentially, the ability to control one's attention is the glue that holds the P3 together.

There are many dimensions to attention, focus, and concentrations across many fields of study including psychology and neuroscience. The term **"attention"** is normally associated with the thoughts or stimuli a person selects to ignore in favor of other thoughts or stimuli that they prefer to apply to their focus. Regardless of whether the stimuli are internal or external, attention is the process that directs one's awareness. The common term **"focus"** is actually a subset component of attention; it is a point at which individuals place their attention in either a broad or narrow perspective, much like the lens of a camera. A person can actively focus on a single item, or passively focus on several items across their environment, but cannot actively and effectively focus on both. Focus represents the direction and clarity of one's attention.

The common term **"concentration"** is another subset component of attention. Concentration is the level of intensity or persistence of focus on a task or object, be it broad or narrow. Essentially, it is the level of energy/effort applied or directed toward one's point of focus. Concentration represents the duration and intensity of one's attention. In other words, it is how long and how deeply a person can sustain focus. Active concentration on a point of focus requires high levels of expended energy whereas passive concentration requires lower levels. Concentration is a skill we all possess to varying degrees, and it can be improved with proper training.

**Attention control** is the level of ability an individual has to selectively control attention on a task. The ability to acquire and sustain appropriate focus and concentration levels are the underlying elements for achieving peak performance in almost every field of work or aspect of life. Without attention control, the simplest tasks become difficult. We all possess the skill to focus on something we choose to attend to, and this skill quickly responds to proper training in practical skills for controlling attention and in achieving the focus and concentration that are essential for elite performances.

World-class performers deal with the same adversity in life as any other person, although high performers seem to be more in tune with certain aspects of their life through **situational awareness** — the ability to size up a situation and make appropriate and timely decisions that contribute to a higher level of performance. Situational awareness is an important aspect of **attentional focus,** as it is an essential contributor to an elite performance level.

**Adaptive thinking** is a conditioned process that uses proven techniques in effective thinking and decision making, performed habitually, to deliver mental toughness and resiliency in the presence of adversity. The conditioning begins with an understanding of cognition and how people attend to their world, the components of memory (recall and recognition), and the establishment of routines and attention (focus) cues designed to engage the subconscious mind to take action in different settings. Spatial cues, for example, can be deep in a person's peripheral field, and with successful recognition of those cues (conditioning similar to the behavioral cues a lifeguard looks for to save lives) a person will habitually respond with desirable behaviors. Elite performers are conditioned to excel because they are adept in the skills listed on the following page.

- Recognizing and prioritizing objectives in adverse high stress situations.
- Developing courses of action development.
- Making decisions.
- Using functional techniques for energy regulation.
- Identifying personal strengths and weaknesses in physical and cognitive abilities, and conducting an assessment to identify personal needs based on this information.
- Identifying the requirement for focus and concentration for a task, and smoothly adjusting to meet those requirements
- Practicing the practical skills that foster a mindset for excellence through the identification of performance objectives, effective thinking habits and management of internal resources, use of cue-initiated routines, and use of mental rehearsal.
- Identifying the psychological factors that affect individual and team performance, and then utilizing the information to create a specific plan of action that meets an individual's or team's performance objectives.
- Developing routines that enable you to navigate successfully through adversity without deviation in performance at a moment when you are forced to act absent the time to analyze properly and prepare.
- Feeling confident in your ability to perform in any adverse situation.

## How Attention Control Is Linked to Elite Performance

Elite performance requires an ability to identify and separate what can and cannot be controlled in order to know where attention should be placed. Likewise, setting goals directs attention to a plan of action that paves the way to a desired outcome. Knowing exactly what to do and how to do it fosters confidence, which neutralizes stressors and conserves or recovers energy. Peak performers know how to direct their attention in a manner that allows them to visualize their performance in different ways. Seeing the technical aspects of a desired outcome in preparation for a significant performance expectation (**preparation mindset**), and broadening the view on an event to allow trust, desire, and a strong belief in themselves enables them to perform cohesively with their environment in order to reach their true potential (**performing mindset**).

One might say that attention control starts by learning to pay attention to one's attention. Peak performers tend to analyze their performances with the purposes of learning in order to improve quickly. Placing a narrow focus on a task, process, position, or technique is the essence of the preparation mindset; however, when it is time to perform, people should not be trying to analyze what they are doing with a deep, narrow focus. Rather, they should be in a softer focus, anticipating adversity (looking for cues) and should trust in their capability to perform based on the work they put into their preparation. True confidence doesn't come from psyching oneself up for a performance; it comes from the work put forth in preparation.

In times of peak performance, a person tends to experience his/her own personal version of "pure focus" — focus in which one's eyes, hands, the entire body act without interference or hesitation to accomplish a task. This is the result of effective focus and concentration. How does one negotiate chaotic city traffic during rush hour? What determines whether a person arrives safely at his/her destination or becomes involved in a collision? It comes down to what one sees, hears, and touches and how the brain manages that information. Professional drivers, regardless of their job, well understand this requirement. Where their focus is at is vital to determining the outcome, whether driving an ambulance, a police car, or a race car, or rolling down the streets looking for improvised explosive devices in a combat zone.

Attention control techniques are essential to help people achieve their performance goals and are an important element of performance excellence. The self-regulation system discussed here can assist a person in becoming aware of how their focus works and how to sustain it. The benefit of an attention control plan is that it helps individuals learn the necessary behaviors that allow concentration to be available when they need it. This is critical to achieving performance excellence in accordance with the performance excellence model.

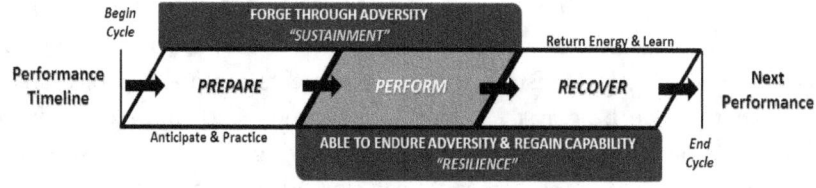

**Performance Excellence Model**

**P3 RESULTS** = Sustainability in higher performance levels in the face of stress and adversity.

The key components of this model are Preparation Strategies, Execution or Performance Sustainment Strategies, and Recovery

88

Strategies. Managing attention is vital in all three components. The skills to prepare for, manage, and recover from intense adversity in order to have increased focus and concentration levels when necessary, are vital to a successful Personal Performance Plan (P3). In order to cope with distractions and become more efficient in adapting to change, one must use effective thinking to identify where focus should be placed and identify the proper level of concentration needed to perform a task and reach true performance potential. A person who is able to master each of the three elements in the self-regulation model can expect to have greater self-awareness, become highly adaptive, and display superior mental agility in the face of adversity.

*Preparation (PREPARE)*. Consistently performing at one's best requires a commitment to preparation. The purposes of preparation are to obtain a mental and physical pre-performance state that anticipates adversity, to establish courses of action to counter it, and to practice those courses of action to ensure successful implementation in accordance with a P3. In fact, preparation is the largest and most comprehensive of the three elements (Prepare, Perform, and Recover) of the P3.

Good preparation includes obtaining appropriate knowledge, mastering techniques and procedures, and preparing the mind and body for demands during the course of a performance. These are essential elements that foster mental toughness. An attention-control plan should be included in the P3 and practiced, ensuring the sustainment of higher levels of performance in the presence of prolonged adversity. The first step to develop an attention-control plan is to identify situations in which one feels distracted and develop a plan to counter those situations. The goal of preparation is to achieve a state of optimal performance readiness which is an essential requirement for consistently superior performances.

*Performance Sustainment (PERFORM)*. Sustaining high levels of performance requires mental toughness and the capacity to recover from and adapt to stress and adversity. Resilience to distraction and recovery of concentration are not just about bouncing back once one's performance levels have dropped. It is just as beneficial to sustain performance levels by preventing obstacles to focus from accumulating during challenging situations or tasks. Trainees can learn how to increase their resilience capacity through practice while preparing to perform. Knowing what to do when adversity strikes is the key to overcoming it. This requires intense conditioning on the skills that are essential for performance excellence. The goal is for responsiveness to be habitual during a performance. Appropriate and timely reactions to demands placed on the mind and body can be the difference between reaching one's performance potential and not performing to expectations.

*Recovery (RECOVER)*. Because focus and concentration are essential for one's survival, a system exists within the mind that monitors levels of focus (broad & narrow) and concentration (energy) to make necessary adjustments in the interest of self-preservation. In humans, as in other higher animals, a system has evolved to take on this responsibility. When a person is in deep concentration for a prolonged period of time as a result of critical thinking, decision making, or in an intense focus for learning, one may begin to feel fatigue setting in. Concentration levels drop because energy reserves devoted to help sustain focus and concentration are becoming depleted. This reaction is the body telling us that our performance capability is diminishing on the task, and if we pay attention to the signs, we will notice the system taking measure to regain energy for concentration. Each demand (stressors or tasks) on the mind or body is different, and each possesses its own requirement of energy in order to achieve a level of optimal functioning. Humans possess distinct parameters for optimal energy levels by task often referred to as "the zone," "zone of optimal performance" or "zone of optimal functioning" where a person performs at potential while expending energy efficiently. In order for people to perform at their best, they must be aware of and be able to monitor their thoughts, behaviors, intensity, and emotions. In order to prepare properly, a person should develop a plan to adjust energy levels to an optimal level anticipating adversity in advance of a performance opportunity or the execution of a task. Techniques for adjusting a person's energy level usually involve some degree of recovery activity at times when the person is experiencing a decline in performance. Muscular tension occurs with anxiety, or over-energy, and interferes with the execution of a person's actions, decreasing optimal performance. Various strategies that foster resilience in focus include specific breathing exercises, such as complete or diaphragmatic breathing, sighing with exhalation, rhythmic breathing and synchronized pattern breathing, and routines that maximize recovery and ensure that attention levels are optimal.

Some people do not view recovery as a priority. They believe that they should be able to endure situations where they are in deep focus for long periods of time. Working late on a project, working double shifts, or long study sessions getting ready for the big exam are just a few of examples of how people sometimes push themselves. They think they are tough enough to push themselves hard and still maintain optimal performance levels; however, science on attention control and energy management tells us something different. Research conducted over the past twenty years proves that there are limits to a person's abilities to focus and concentrate. Most colleges, technical schools, and even junior levels of education organize their classes to last 50 minutes and include a 10 minute break. These changes were made as a result of compelling research conducted in the 1970s reflecting human capability to sustain focus using concentration in a demanding academic (study) environment. These lessons are now considered "rules" for learning and can be applied to other aspects of life. Regardless of profession, one should acknowledge and become aware of attention requirements for performing critical tasks and use and practice the proper attention-control techniques discussed in this program. Proper focus and concentration are necessary to push a person to reach performance potential. High levels of prolonged exposure to tough and demanding situations involving intense narrow focus that is not regulated properly can be detrimental to sustaining peak performance levels.

## Train Like a World Class Performer

Everything covered in this training program contributes to world-class performances in different ways. Whether a person applies the lessons to work performance, athletic performance, academic performance, or some other area of life such as health-care regimens, it is vital to understand how to incorporate lessons learned into a personal or team performance plan. How these techniques are incorporated into professional and Olympic athletics performance plans and in U.S. Military Special Forces training can be useful in developing individual performance plans.

One of the most critical elements of superior performance is "controlling one's attention." Superior performances depend largely on one's ability to focus and concentrate properly during the course of execution of a task or performance situation. Where trainees place their focus will determine how quickly they learn new information and techniques associated with a task and condition themselves for psychomotor habitual responsiveness which increases reaction times and helps the performer navigate adversity under the most demanding conditions. How trainees manage their attention directly contributes to how they feel about themselves going into a performance (positively or negatively). Careful attention management, energy management, and thoughtful decision making all contribute to the confidence trainees will have as they face high levels of demand.

*Attention Training for Military Special Forces.* On November 16, 2004, an NBC News cameraman filmed a U.S. Marine killing an unarmed and wounded insurgent in a Mosque in Fallujah, Iraq. The film footage of this event seemed to show that a war crime had been committed. This was big news for about two weeks until it faded away without coverage of the outcome. What most people do not know about this event is that the Marine in question was cleared of any wrong-doing due to the incident being considered a "poor decision" the marine made in the heat of battle and not a war crime. Most people close to the case considered it closed; however, the Army Special Operations Command began to ask a couple of questions that would end up changing the way U.S. military Special Forces train. The questions were, "How could the military train someone to make the right decision in a situation like that?" and "Is the Army conditioning service members to make life and death mistakes?" Elements at the United States Military Academy at West Point, the Army Center for

Enhanced Performance, the JFK Special Warfare Center and School, and the Army research lab worked together with elements of the Joint Special Operations Command to answer these questions, and to come up with a better way to train.

The outcome of the investigation revealed that conventional training methods conditioned service members to perform toward a specific conclusion. Mistakes normally occurred when the conditions surrounding an event were not the same as the conditions for which the service member was trained. It was clear that conventional training methods did not prepare service members with the skill to adapt to variation, and in many cases, it was actually counterproductive. Put simply, investigators began to realize that service members were actually being conditioned to make mistakes. Because of these investigations and others like it in and out of the Department of Defense, techniques in adaptive thinking quickly became the focus in modern training.

**Conditioning with Cues and Routines**

In order for a person to react to high-stress situations, the human brain quickly reaches for information in the effort to help them assess the situation, analyze courses of action, prepare their body and thoughts to respond, and finally to take some kind of action in response to the demands of the situation. When service members train, they are given a task to perform, they examine the conditions under which they will be asked to perform, and then they are given the performance standards for which they will be evaluated. This all sounds clear enough; however, once the training begins they are exposed to tremendous adversity, forcing their attention to be shared by many points of focus, the idea being that they would learn to cope with the adversity due to repeated exposure. Perhaps the biggest flaw in conventional military training is that it does not have sufficient respect for how human memory works. One thing conventional military training does is stress the use of "**Recall**" to retrieve information from the brain enabling them to respond to a demand. As previously discussed, recall is redundant conditioning of an action or routine to strengthen neural pathways to the point where the service member will respond habitually in a situation. This is a process known as "**neuroplasticity**," wherein a person is constantly exposed to demands, and the mind and body respond to help the person meet those demands. Neuroplasticity is a common treatment for reconditioning the brain in response to trauma, such as Traumatic Brain Injury, Alzheimer's, and other brain injuries or degenerative conditions.

Neuroplasticity works well to condition a person to respond; however, there is no guarantee that the person will respond correctly regardless of how much training he/she has. The problem is that no training scenario can exactly match what happens in the real world. If trainees are not conditioned with a "**recognition**" cue along with the recall, they are forced to rely on their ability to think critically about the situation (conscious response rather than a habitual response) in order to know when and how to respond. This slows reaction times considerably, requiring a person to analyze and decide on a course of action and make a decision before reacting. If the person does not have the proper time to do all that, then the person is much more likely to make a mistake. In the Marine example, the service member was conditioned to enter and clear a room in accordance with a preset drill in order to secure it. The service member's training involved a violent entry, aggressive maneuver to a point of domination in the room, and engaging the enemy with his weapon as required. This Marine likely did this same drill hundreds of times in training, and the controversial video showed him doing the same. The conclusions were that the Marine did exactly what he was conditioned to do. Why would anyone think he would respond differently? Without conditioning with clear recognition cues to tell him when to react habitually, the service member is forced to make a hasty decision to engage or not to engage; kill or not to kill. The Marine made a mistake because of his conditioning through conventional training.

## Mental Circuit Training

Today, Army Special Forces Soldiers and Navy Seals train with recognition cues emphasized. This approach is consistent with how world class Olympic athletes and some athletes from professional sports have trained for over ten years. It is beneficial to dissect a task down to its lowest required skill, and then identify cues that will support activation of those skills for task completion. These cues are then conditioned to a point where the person responds to them habitually without the need for thoughts or conscious decisions to be made. Some Army Special Forces teams at Fort Bragg, North Carolina refer to this type of conditioning as "**mental circuit training**" because they would engage in this activity immediately after their physical training which often included physical strength and conditioning circuits. Many players in the National Football League view it similarly. As soldiers would use these techniques to respond to a threat, NFL players use it to react to an opponent. Business executives use these techniques to mitigate risk by establishing operating boundaries (cues) to protect against waste and poor decision-making.

If the Marine discussed in the earlier example had been training correctly back in 2004, he would have been conditioned to respond to cues such as the raising of a weapon in a threatening manner as a recognition cue to respond with a routine conditioned with recall. This would have allowed him to turn and engage the enemy habitually if the situation called for it, or not engage in favor of another routine designed to contain an unarmed and wounded person. Either action would have been accomplished without the need for further analyzing because the correct conditions (cues) existed to allow deadly force to be initiated if a legitimate threat existed. If the conditions (cues) are not

93

presented, then the service member would react by using conscious thought and critical thinking to analyze courses of action before reacting or making a decision. If he had been trained this way, he would not have to live the rest of his life knowing that a person lost his life because he made a mistake. This is arguably one of the greatest fears of law enforcement officers and armed security personnel today.

## Learning from the Military

Lessons learned and changes made in military training have captured the attention of world-class athletes and elite business executives. The concept of reacting decisively and correctly to adversity may translate differently in value depending on the field, but the conditioning process for achieving positive outcome is pretty much the same. Many athletes and coaches from the U.S. Olympic Training Center visit the U.S. military to study methods they feel will help them reach a higher level of performance in their sport. Professional athletes from many sports are also interested in cutting-edge performance enhancement techniques the military uses to train and condition service members. One such military program that is frequently visited is the Center for Enhanced Performance at the United States Military Academy at West Point. This unique work unit has the specific mission of continuously gathering the latest science and best practices in the field of human performance. Relentless pursuit of performance excellence has also attracted business executives looking to improve processes and boost productivity while reducing costs in an ever-changing environment filled with adversity.

It does not matter if it is in the world of business, athletics, law enforcement, or the military, the mechanics behind how a person pays attention are pretty much the same, and the process for improving focus and dealing with distractions is also the same. The differences lie in the conditions surrounding a performance and the level of adversity one faces. If a person wishes to raise his/her performances and sustain high levels of functioning in the face of adversity, the first thing to do is to "**pay attention to how you pay attention**."

Selected references are presented here for readers who may wish to pursue greater understanding of the research and science behind performance excellence.

Amen, D. (2005). *Making a Good Brain Great*

Anderson, J. R. (2000). *Learning and Memory: An Integrated Approach*.

Anshel, M. (2007). *Conceptualizing Applied Exercise Psychology*

Butler & Hope. (2007). *Managing Your Mind: the Mental Fitness Guide*

Carlson, Neil R. (2010). *Psychology: The Science of Behavior*.

Conrad, C.D. (2010). *A Critical Review of Chronic Stress Effects on Spatial Learning and Memory*

Cowan, N. (2001). *The Magical Number 4 in Short-term Memory: A Reconsideration of Mental Storage Capacity*

Deagle, Henegham & Raybourn. (2005). *Adaptive Thinking & Leadership: Simulation Game Training for Special Forces Officers*

Demos, J. (2004). *Getting Started in Neurofeedback*

LaBar & Cabeza. (2006). *Cognitive Neuroscience of Emotional Memory*

Mills, K. (2005). *Disciplined Attention*

Ratey, J. (2002). *A User's Guide to the Brain*

Ruesch, J. E. (2011). *Controlling Your Attention*

Schwabe & Wolf (2010). *Learning Under Stress Impairs Memory Formation*

Van Blerkom, D. L. (2011). *College Study Skills: Becoming a Strategic Learner*

Voorhies, D. (2004). *Adaptive Leadership: The Creative Application of Battle Command*

Additional/Special Contributions: Jarvin Heiman, MD. Lecture on Brain Science, 2000

# Leadership Challenges

For decades, researchers have examined leadership and the inspiration that successful leaders can create in their efforts to transform people, cultures, and performance and to build healthy teams and organizations. The results of such research suggest that transformational leaders exhibit and cultivate enthusiasm and can inject passion and energy into people who are willing to collaborate. They can motivate people to change at a fast pace when a vision is communicated and trust is engendered. A faith alliance is generated when stakeholders believe that the transformational leader's plan will work — a vision that is reinforced as conviction and commitment grow throughout an organization.

In their book *Every Officer Is a Leader* (2012), Dr. Terry Anderson and colleagues provide a model to build a "leadership and learning organization" in order to diminish organizational stress and to optimize team and organizational performance for the benefit of both the organization and the larger community. According to their Transforming Leadership Model, a leadership organization prepares leaders first. Eventually everyone who works *in* the organization works *on* it (to improve it). People begin to see their individual contributions in the context of the organization as a whole if they are given feedback about their contributions. They are enlightened as they see how their work influences internal and external interactions and outcomes. They are aligned with reality when they understand how their decisions and actions are contributing to the service quality of the organization. It is clear that a leadership organization is not ordinary, nor is it subject to a quick and simple transition; but it is perhaps a necessity if the goal is to move forward into a preferred future. The chart on the following page offers a comparison of traditional organizational characteristics and the key attributes of a leadership organization.

| Traditional Organization | Leadership Organization |
| --- | --- |
| Controls organizational design | Is co-designed by those who work in it |
| Assumes it knows what is best | Assumes that what is best is always changing |
| Delays change as long as possible | Responds to change immediately |
| Clings to old paradigms | Anticipates change in advance whenever possible |
| Applies a linear approach | Uses a systems approach |
| Uses vertical command hierarchies | Develops collegial team relationships |
| Sees work as boring repetition | Sees work as meaningful self-expression |
| Sees people as cogs in wheels | Sees people as collaborators, teammates |
| Focuses on past and present | Focuses on moving toward ideal future |
| Is sufficiency-oriented | Is continuous-improvement oriented |
| Is bureaucracy-oriented | Is people- and idea-oriented |
| Manages by objectives | Applies strategic, accountable, intuitive leadership |
| Respects traditional gender roles | Recognizes, rewards competency |
| Has multiple levels in organizational structure | Cross-functions through information access and role clarity |
| Manages by position power | Leads by credibility |
| Attacks problems | Processes or prevents problems |
| Conforms to rules | Uses creative problem-solving for continuous improvement |
| Does decision-making out of | Uses inter-team brainstorming and consultation decision- making |
| Is accountable to the boss | Is accountable to the team |
| Has a self-interest orientation | Respects quality and customer service orientation |
| Results are top priority at all costs | Intelligent, creative people produce more results and build people at the same time |
| Rewards those who conform | Rewards people based on their ability to help achieve strategic objectives |

The skills outlined in the Leadership Organization are offered to leaders for the development of effective team and organizational performance, but leaders need to be free of the personality problems that cause nearly half of them to derail. In a meta-analysis of the studies that reveal the primary causes of management derailment, members of the Hogan Assessment System (Hogan, et al., 2009) found that nearly half of leaders internationally and across multiple sectors have consistently failed to be effective. They assert that leaders not only need to understand leadership but also need to learn competencies that support and enhance the promise of success. While the root causes of leadership failure are more complex than simply the one factor of personality, it is a factor that cannot be ignored, as the Hogan team notes:

> The behaviors associated with managerial derailment are well documented and are relevant to most organizations and most managers. . . . The "dark side" personality factors help explain why managers have relationship problems. The derailment research also points to the role of change, stress, and a lack of self-awareness as potentiating factors. The research leads to some useful generalizations, offers taxonomies of causes and early warning signals, and remedial recommendations.

Thus, if organizational health and wellness are to be taken seriously, it is important that key decision-makers take leadership development and personality seriously when selecting, orienting, training, supervising, and promoting leaders. The Hogan organization offers a suite of psychological assessments that clarify root causes of most of the disorders and that encourage careful and thorough consideration of the factors that may predict performance or may cause managers to derail at some point in their career. Additional information about such assessments is available at the website: www.HoganAssessments.com

***Transforming Leadership: A Research- and Philosophy-based Model.*** There are so many theories and philosophical assumptions about what leaders should do to become more effective that it may be difficult to distinguish the panaceas from thoughtful research- and practice-based programs. The concepts and leadership skill sets in the Transforming Leadership model (please see the graphics on the next page) are based on applicable research and theory in self-mastery, interpersonal communication, counseling, coaching, mentoring, consulting, organization development, and human resource development. The model is backed by numerous practical examples of how each skill can be applied in concert with other skills to form a comprehensive approach to the development of people, teams, and organizations. As a result, they can make a positive impact on the security and safety of communities.

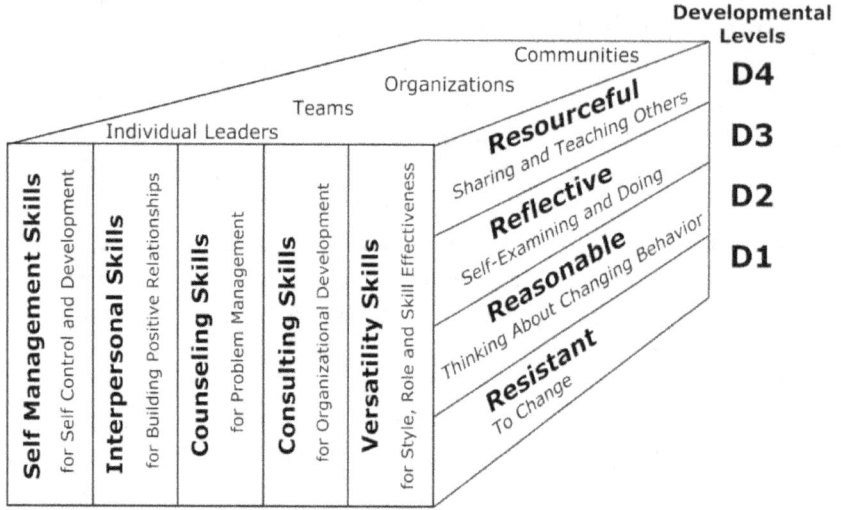

**Five Transforming Leadership Skill Sets**

Law enforcement leaders who utilize the leadership skill sets and knowledge areas in the model have greater potential to shape organizational climate and the interpersonal environment to achieve desired strategic and operational results that can so powerfully build and protect communities. Moreover, organizational learning and organizational health go hand in hand, and the model provides for learning assessments that are varied and comprehensive. It is not at all surprising that a mindful, conscientious leadership organization reduces organizational and individual stress and thereby improves health throughout the organization.

At first glance, it may appear that the leadership model presented here is not immediately applicable to law enforcement agencies in which hierarchical structures have traditionally dominated. Nevertheless, police agencies that have successfully embraced community policing may have a head-start, albeit a rough one, in the difficult task of structuring their agencies to meet the constantly changing and rapidly accelerating demands of their communities. Leaders in those agencies have found that creating rapport and building trust and cooperation are critical elements in building a healthy and resilient police force in which shared goals are communicated openly and energetically.

Clearly, a major goal in any law enforcement agency is to maintain a healthy and resilient workforce, but it is unlikely that such a goal can be reached unless the stigma of reporting stress-related illness can be eradicated. An anonymous letter from an urban police sergeant makes the point: " I love my work . . . [but] I can't sleep at night and my belly goes crazy when things heat up at work. My career is important to me and my family, and I don't dare get help because I can't let anyone know that I'm sick. Maybe I'm not sick, just stressed."

The denial of need is a crucible for an epidemic, and the directive for law enforcement leadership is obvious. In an exuberant learning environment, police agency leaders have the opportunity to effectively understand and diminish mental-health challenges of peace officers. The communities they serve likewise have such responsibilities and opportunities.

### Organizational Health

"A resilient police organization makes the difference," according to Dr. John Violanti (n.d.) writing in *The Jimston Journal* about law enforcement organizational climate, trust, and leadership. It is the police organization, he maintains, that creates the framework against which officers experience, interpret, and define their work and establish performance patterns in which capabilities are nurtured or curtailed. Officers' perceptions of how their organization functions are the molds in which their roles and actions in the organization are set. Clearly, police agencies have a key role in facilitating officer performance, adaptability, and resilience, and according to Dr. Violanti, organizational climate is a major influence on officers' ability to positively meet the challenges of critical-incident experiences. Positive work cultures have a direct and positive effect on coping success.

Peace officers are not particularly noted for an inclination to trust, perhaps because trust may be associated with vulnerability on the street, perhaps even because of work experiences that reward an officer's ability to discern falsehoods and sidestep dangers. Nevertheless, trust is a major determinant in effective group processes, interpersonal relationships, and organizational efficacy, and lack of trust may obstruct officers' willingness to seek assistance when necessary. Trust also supports authentic empowerment and meaning and is associated with adaptability and capacity to deal effectively with complex, high-risk events. Law enforcement leaders who successfully negotiate the challenges of high-stress environments understand that openness and trust foster opportunities for learning and for mutual, cooperative well-being.

Attentive leadership draws away from an officer's personal and psychological preoccupations and creates an environment of shared responsibility, mutual respect, and cohesion. Leaders translate organizational culture into reliable policies, processes, and values that sustain officers. Under caring and competent leadership, resilience forms naturally and organically and can be nurtured to shape confidence, integrity, and opportunity throughout the organization.

### Maintaining Learning Environments

Police officers entering their service careers engage in demanding and effective training. Sadly, the specters of fatigue and funding may thereafter diminish enthusiasm for learning or derail opportunities for personal or organizational growth, awareness, and effectiveness. In his book on *Futuring: The Exploration of the Future,*

101

Edward Cornish puts habituated lethargy and resistance to change into a challenging perspective.

> We are all time travellers on a journey into the future . . . explorers in an unknown and dangerous region. . . . Reading accounts of great expeditions we notice that [past] explorers prepared very carefully for their expeditions. Their success depended on having the right equipment, the right supplies, the right teammates, and the right training at the moment of need. . . . [R]esources that can help us deal with the unexpected include a good understanding of our changing world, intellectual tools for thinking ahead, and methods for assessing our options.
>
> *Edward Cornish is founder and former president of the World Future Society and editor of its magazine,* The Futurist.

The accumulation of knowledge that occurs over time has formed a massive, retrievable knowledge base that continues to grow each day, each hour. Mr. Cornish makes the point that 80 percent of all scientists who have ever lived are alive today. It is not a spectator sport, this *life* thing; you have to be present to be present. With learning, many things are possible, and the 21st century peace officer must be free to think critically and openly, to adapt and perform using innovation and novel concepts and traditional "go to" habits alike.

We turn to the 14th Dalai Lama for another perspective on the leadership challenges and the benefits of creating and maintaining learning environments:

> Education is the best way to train ourselves that we will secure our own well-being by concerning ourselves with others. It is  possible to create a better world, a more compassionate, more  peaceful world, which is not only in everyone's interest, but is  everyone's responsibility to achieve.
>
> Tenzin Gyatso, His Holiness the Fourteenth Dalai Lama Reprinted from *Change Your Mind, Change the World - Discussion to Make the World a Healthier, Happier Place* (May, 2013). ww.dalailama.com/news/post/947-change-your-mind-change-the-world---discussion-to-make-the-world-a-healthier-happier-place

# Onward

In his book, *The Better Angels of Our Nature: Why Violence Has Declined*, Harvard Professor Steven Pinker outlines global trends over the past several hundred years that indicate a decrease in human violence. He presents an optimistic trajectory of hope for mankind as we enter perhaps the most complex era in our history. Likewise, as we have reviewed pathways to wellness and resilience, based on both vision and science, we have sought healing and hope for those who serve as protectors of life.

Many cultures throughout human history held the belief that the sun influenced their activities and behaviors, and of course they were correct. Sunlight and seasonal weather cycles are inevitably interwoven with food supplies and thus with survival and even the flourishing of all life. Today, we often appear to be fluctuating between sun worship and sunscreen as we attempt to adapt to the accelerating speed of change. We look to scientists and philosophers to map the rising temperature of the future and make it understandable.

Organizations such as the Institute of HeartMath offer a wealth of information. If, as they suspect, violence, crime rate, social unrest, revolutions, and frequency of terrorist attacks are linked to the solar cycle and the resulting disturbances in the geomagnetic field, are we then little more than hostage organisms on a planet that may go out of control at any moment? Likely not. The Institute points out that solar activity is also related to periods of human flourishing in the arts and sciences and in positive social evolution. John Steinbeck suggested that "we must look from the tidepool to the stars and back again."

We must look inward (the tidepool) and discover or rediscover that conscience is awareness of mindful and moral conduct and that fidelity to a worthy purpose is the truest and most ethical ambition — the one most likely to support the well-being of us all. Individually and collectively on a global scale, we can embrace the HeartMath conclusion that living systems are interconnected and communicate with each other by way of biological and electromagnetic fields, giving us just cause to celebrate: Humans can decide to work together to consciously increase coherence in the global field environment and thus in their countries, their communities, and in themselves. The natural flow of human consciousness is heart-based, learning-based—hinging on cooperation not competition— and bathed in empathy and compassion.

Research conducted during the first decade of the twenty-first century was unusually rich for individuals and agencies attempting to understand the complexities of human interactions and to consider how they might constructively influence outcomes. Police officers are becoming increasingly aware of how their attitudes and behaviors are significant determinants of outcome in both stressful and benign encounters. As we have seen in this work, attitudes and behaviors are likewise significant determinants of good health. We may elect to see ourselves as victims of a particular illness, but clearly we must see ourselves as responsible participants in our recovery. And we must ask our law enforcement leaders and our communities to share responsibility for eradicating stigmas associated with illness, especially illness that may be a wound acquired in the line of duty.

Throughout this work, we have used the terms "peace officer" and "police officer" interchangeably and with gratitude for all officers who are called to stand in that place of risk as protectors of life and promoters of peace. The vote has not yet been tallied with regard to which term may prevail, and it may be that learning — free from habituated thinking or from preoccupations that are disabling or obsolete — will determine our evolutionary path toward the co-creation of a more positive and intentional future. Today is the day to celebrate the possibility that cooperation, empathy, altruism, critical thinking, ethical behavior, and good health will be the biomarkers of our accelerating psychophysiological evolution. Our celebration honors the many peace-officer heroes who dare to care for self and others.

# References

The extensive citations in the text of *Beyond Survival Tactics* are included for the benefit of readers who may wish to further pursue the rich history of scholarship relating to law enforcement and to human well-being

Akers, R. L. (2009). *Social learning and social structure: A general theory of crime and deviance.* New Brunswick, NJ: Transaction Publishers.

American Psychological Association (2011). Stress and gender. Retrieved from www.apa.org/news/press/releases/stress/2011/gender.aspx and www.apa.org/news/press/releases/stress/gender-stress.aspx

Anderson, T., Gisborne, K., Holliday, P. (2012). Every officer is a leader : Coaching leadership, learning and performance in justice, public safety, and security organizations. Indianapolis, IN: Trafford Publishing

Andrew, M.E, McCanlies, E.C., Burchfiel, C.M., Charles, L.E., Hartley, T.A., Fekedulegn, D., & Violanti, J.M. (2008). Hardiness and psychological distress in a cohort of police officers. *International Journal of Emergency Mental Health, 10*(2), 137-147.

Arroyo-Morales. M, Olea, N., Martinez, M., Moreno-Lorenzo, C., Díaz-Rodríguez , L., & Hidalgo-Lozano, A.(2008). Effects of myofascial release after high-intensity exercise: a randomized clinical trial, *Journal of Manipulative Physiological Therapy. 31*(3),217–23.

Asmundson, G.J., & Stapleton, J. A. (2008). Associations between dimensions of anxiety sensitivity and PTSD symptoms clusters in active-duty police officers. *Cognitive Behavior Therapy, 37*(2), 66-75. doi: 10.1080/16506070801969005

Azar, B. (2000). A new stress paradigm for women. *American Psychological Association Monitor, 32*(7), 42. Retrieved from

Barnes, J., Phillipson, J.D., & Anderson, L.A. ( 2007). *Herbal medicines,* 3rd ed. Produced under the direction of the Royal Pharmaceutical Society of Great Britain. London, UK: Pharmaceutical Press.

Bernard, L. C., & Krupat, E. (1994). *Health psychology: Biopsychosocial factors in health and illness.* New York: Harcourt Brace College Publishers.

Bradley, R.A., McCraty, R., Lash, M, & Laraway, L. (2011) The coherence advantage: Resilience mentoring field guide. Boulder Creek, C A: Institute of Heart Math.

Calaprice, A. (Ed.). (2000). *The Expanded Quotable Einstein.* Princeton, N J: Princeton University Press.

Chopko, B. (2010). Posttraumatic stress and growth: An empirical study of police officers. *American Journal of Psychotherapy, 64*(1), 55-72.

Chopko, B., & Schwartz, R. C. (2009). The relationship between mindfulness and posttraumatic growth: A study of first responders to trauma-inducing incidents. *Journal of Mental Health Counseling, 31*(4), 363-376.

Colvin, H.M.,& Taylor, R.M., R*apporteurs* (2012). *Building a resilient workforce: Opportunities for the Department of Homeland Security: Workshop summary, Board on Health Sciences Policy: Institute of Medicine.* Washington DC: The National Academies Press.

Cornish, E. (2004) *Futuring: The exploration of the future.* Bethesda, MD: World Future Society.

Dale, R.A.*(2005). Tao Te Ching: A new translation and commentary.* New York, NY: Fall River Press.

Daniels,. D.L. (2008). Post-traumatic stress disorder and the causal link to crime: A looming national tragedy (Doctoral dissertation, United States Army) retrieved from http://www.dtic.mil/cgi-bin/GETTRDoc.pdf.

Dokoupil, T. (2012). A new theory of PTSD and veterans: Moral injury. Retrieved from **www.**thedailybeast.com/newsweek/2012/12/02/a-new-theory-of-ptsd-and-veterans-moral-injury.html.

Dorfman, D.N. (1999). Proving the lie: Litigating police credibility. *American Journal of Criminal Law, 26*(3), 455-503.

Du, J., Wang, Y., Hunter, R., Wei, Y., Blumenthal, R., Falke, C., Khairova, R.., Zhou, R., Yuan, P., Machado-Vieira, R., McEwen, B.S., & Manji, H.K. (2009). Dynamic regulation of mitochondrial function by glucocorticoids. *Proceedings of the National Academy of Sciences of the United States,. 106*(9), 3543-3548. doi: 10.1073/pnas.0812671106

Elbogen, E. G., Johnson, S.C., Wagner, H. R.. , Newtown, V. M., & Beckman, J. C. (2012). Financial well-being and post deployment adjustment among Iraq and Afghanistan war veterans. *Military Medicine 177*(6) 669-675.

Erneling, C. E., & Johnson, D. M. (Eds.). (2004). *Mind as a scientific object: Between brain and culture.* Cary, NC: Oxford University Press.

Engbeck, J. (2011). *Patrol services for crime-free communities: Methods, procedures, alliance, and integration.* ISBN 13: 978-1466257344.

Fabricant, D.S. & Farnsworth, N.R. (2001). The value of plants used in traditional medicine for drug discovery. *Environmental Health Perspectives, 109*(supplement 1), 69-75.

Ford, J.K., (2007). Building capability throughout a change effort: Leading the transformation of a police agency to community policing. *American Journal of Community Psychology, 39,* 3-4, 321–334.

Ford, J.K., Weissbein, D., & Plammondon, K. (2003). Distinguishing organizational commitment from strategy commitment: Linking officer commitment to community policing to work behaviors and job satisfaction. *Justice Quarterly, 20* (1), 159-185.

Franke, W.D., Kohut, M.L., Russell, D.W., Yoo, H.L., Ekkekakis, P., & Ramey, S.L. (2010). Is job-related stress the link between cardiovascular disease and the law enforcement profession? *Journal of Occupational & Environmental Medicine 52*(5), 561-565. doi: 10.1097/JOM.0b013e3181dd086b

Franken, R.E. (1994). *Human Motivation,* 3rd ed. Belmont, CA: Brooks/Cole Publishing Company.

Garbarino, S., Chiorri, C., Magnavita, N., Piattino, S., & Cuomo, G. (2012a). Personality profiles of special force police officers. *Journal of Police and Criminal Psychology, 27*(2), 99-110. doi: 10.1007/s11896-011-9099-6

Garbarino, S., Magnavita, N., Chiorri, C., Brisinda, D., Cuomo, G., Venuti, A., & Fenici, R. (2012b). Evaluation of operational stress in riot and crowd control police units: A global challenge for prevention and management of police task-related stress. *Journal of Police and Criminal Psychology,(27)*2, 111-122. doi:10.1007/s11896-012-9104-8

Gell-Mann, M. (Producer). (2010). Beauty and truth in physics. Retrieved from www. ted.com/talks/murray_gell_mann_on_beauty_and_truth_in_physics.html.

Gershon, R.R.M, Barocas, B., Canton, A.N., Li, X, & Vlahov, D. (2009). Mental, physical, and behavioral outcomes associated with perceived work stress in police officers. *Criminal Justice and Behavior, 36*(3), *275-289.*

Gilmartin, K.M. (2002). *Emotional survival for law enforcement: A guide for officers and their families.* Tucson, AZ: E-S Press. ISBN 0971725403

Goleman, D. & Gyatso, T. (2003*). Destructive emotions: A dialogue with the Dalai Lama.* New York, NY: Bantam Dell.

Goleman, D. & Gyatso, T. (2003*). Healing emotions: Conversations with the Dalai Lama on mindfulness, emotions, and health* Boston, MA: Shambhala Publications.

Green, B. (2009). Problem-based psychiatry (2nd ed.) Oxford, UK: Radcliffe Publishing.

Greubel, J., & Kecklund, G. (2011). The impact of organizational changes on work stress, sleep, recovery and health. *Industrial Health,49*(3), 353-364.

Groer, M., Murphy, R.. Bunnell, W., Saloman, K., Van Eepoel, J., Rankin, B., White, K., & Bykowski, C. (2010). Salivary measures of stress and immunity in police officers engaged in simulated critical incident scenarios. *Journal of Occupational and Environmental Medicine, 52*(6), 592-602.

Grossman, P., Nieman, L., Schmidt, S., & Walach, H. (2004). Mindfulness-based stress reduction and health benefits. *Journal of Psychosomatic Research, 57*(1), 35-43.

Grundy, S.M. (2008). Metabolic syndrome pandemic. *Arteriosclerosis, Thrombosis, and Vascular Biology. 28*, 629-636. doi: 10.1161/ TVBAHA.107.151092

Gyatso, T. & Cutler, H.C. (1998). *The art of happiness: A handbook for living.* New York, NY: Riverhead Books.

Hawkins, D.R. (2012, revised edition). *Power vs. force: The hidden determinants of human behavior.* Carlsbad, CA: Hayhouse

Heal, C. (2012) *Field command.* Lantern Books, Kindle Edition.

HeartMath. (2012). Coherence advantage: Building stress resistance and optimizing performance. Institute of HeartMath. Retrieved from http://www.heartmath.org/training/military/active-duty.html

Hickman, M.J., Fricas, J., Strom, K.J., and Pope, M.W. (2011). Mapping police stress. *Police Quarterly, 14(*3).227-250. doi: 10.1177/1098611111413991

Hink, J. (2010). The returning military veteran: Is your organization ready? *FBI Law Enforcement Bulletin.* Retrieved from

http://www.fbi.gov/stats-services/publications/law-
enforcement-bulletin/august-2010/the-returning-military-veteran.

Hogan, J., Hogan, R., & Kaiser, R. (2009). Management derailment:
Personality assessment and mitigation. Sheldon Zedeck (Editor).
*American Psychological Association of Industrial and Organizational
Psychology*. Washington, DC: American Psychological Association.

Horowitz, M, Wilner, N., & Alvarez W. (1979). Impact of Event Scale: A
measure of subjective stress. *Psychosomatic Medicine* 41(3) 209-218.

Joseph, N.P., Violanti, J.M., Donahue, R., Andrew, M.E., Trevisan, M.,
Burchfiel, C.M., & Dorn, J. (2009). Police work and subclinical
atherosclerosis. *Journal of Occupational and Environmental Health*, *51*(6),
700-707. doi: 10.1097/JOM.0b013e3181a02252

Kabat-Zinn, J., Massion, A.O., Kristeller, J., Peterson, L.G., Fletcher,
K.E., Pbert, L. Lenderking, W.R., & Santorelli, S.F. (1992).
Effectiveness of a meditation-based stress reduction program in the
treatment of anxiety disorders. *The American Journal of Psychiatry 149*(7)
936-43.

Kabat-Zinn, J. & Davidson, R. (2012). *The* m*ind's own physician: A scientific
dialogue with the Dalai Lama on the healing power of meditation*. Oakland,
CA: New Harbinger Publications.

Kloog, I., Portnov, B.A., Rennert, H.S., & Haim, A. (2011). Does the
modern urbanized sleeping habitat pose a breast cancer risk?
*Chronobiology International*, 28(1), 76-80.
doi: 10.3109/07420528.2010.531490

Koo, J.A., & Duman, R.S. (2008). IL-1β is an essential mediator of the
antineurogenic and anhedonic effects of Stress. *Proceedings of the
National Academy of sciences of the United States of America*,*105* (2) 751-
756. doi: 0.1073/pnas.0708092105

Lambert, E. (2007). A test of a turnover intent model: The issue of
correctional staff satisfaction and commitment. In D. E. Duffee and
E. R. Maguire (Eds). *Criminal Justice Theory: Explaining the Nature and
Behavior of Criminal Justice*. New York, NY: Routledge

Lambert, E., & Hogan, N.( 2006). A test of model of turnover intent
among correctional staff at a Midwestern private prison. Paper
presented at the annual meeting of the American Society of
Criminology (ASC), Los Angeles Convention Center. Retrieved from
www.allacademic.com/meta/p114872_index.html.

Levitin, D.J. (2006). This is your brain on music: The science of human
obsession: human nature. New York, NY: Dutton/Penguin.

Levitin, D.J. (2008). The world in six songs: How the musical brain created
human nature. New York, NY: Dutton/Penguin.

Lindauer, R.J.L, Olff, M., van Meijel, E.P.M., Carlier, I.V.E., & Gersons,
B.P.R. (2006). Cortisol, learning, memory, and attention in relation
to smaller hippocampal volume in police officers with
posttraumatic stress disorder. *Biological Psychiatry*, *59(*2), 171-177.

Litz, B.T., Stein, N., Delaney, E., Lebowitz, L., Nash, W.P., Silva, C., &
Maguen, S. (2009). Moral injury and moral repair in war veterans: A
preliminary model and intervention strategy. *Clinical Psychology
Review*,*29*(8):695-706. doi:10.1016/j.cpr.2009.07.003

Marmar, C.R., McCaslin, S.E., Metzler, T.J., Best S., Weiss, D.S., Fagan, J., Liberman, A., Pole, N., Otte, C., Yehuda, R., Mohr, D., & Neylan, T. (2006). Predictors of posttraumatic stress in police and other first responders. *Annals of the New York Academy of Sciences, 1071*(1) 1–18. doi: 10.1196/annals.1364.001

Marquart, J.W., Barnhill, M.B., & Balshaw-Biddle, K. (2001). Fatal attraction: An analysis of employee boundary violations in a southern prison system, 1995-1998. *Justice Quarterly, 18*(4), 877-910.

McCarty, W.P., Zhao, J.S., & Garland, B.E. (2007). Occupational stress and burnout between male and female police officers: Are there any gender differences? *Policing: An International Journal of Police Strategies & Management 39*(4), *672-691. doi:* 10.1108/13639510710833938

McCraty, R.., & Tomasino, D.( 2006). Emotional stress, positive emotions, and psychophysiological coherence. In, *Stress in Health and Disease.* Bengt B. Arnetz & Rolf Ekman, editors. Wiley-VCH, Weinheim.

McCraty, R., Atkinson, Tomasino, & Bradley (2006).The coherent heart: Heart-brain interactions, psychophysiological coherence, and the emergence of system-wide order. E-Book, The Institute of HeartMath. http://www.heartmath.org/research/research-library/research-library.html

McCraty, R., Atkinson, M., Lipsenthal, L., & Arguelles, L. (2009). New hope for correctional officers: An innovative program for reducing stress and health risks. *Applied Psychophysiology and Biofeedback, 34*(4):251-72. doi: 10.1007/s10484-009-9087-0..

McCraty, R., Deyhle, A., & Childre, D. (2012). The global coherence initiative: Creating a coherent planetary standing wave. *Global Advances in Health and Medicine, 1*(1), 64-77. www.gahmj.com

McCrae, R.R. & John, O.P. (1992). An introduction to the five-factor model and its applications. *Journal of Personality 60*(2), 175-215. *doi:* 10.1111/j.1467-6494.1992.tb00970.x

Melchizedek, D. (1999 and 2000)). *The ancient secret of the flower of life, Vols. 1 and 2).* Flagstaff, AZ: Light Technology Publishing.

Miller, L. (2012). *Criminal psychology: Nature, nurture, culture: A textbook and practical reference guide for students and working professionals in the fields of law enforcement, criminal justice, mental health, and forensic psychology.* Springfield, IL: Charles C. Thomas Publisher.

Moira, A. (1999). *Green witchcraft: Folk magic, fairy lore, and herb craft.* St. Louis, MO: Llewellyn Publishing.

Mrazek, D. (2011). Stress, genetics can trigger depression.  Retrieved from http://www.mayoclinic.com/health/stress-and-depression/MY01649.

Nelson, M.C. & Ruiz, M. A. (1997). *Beyond fear: A Toltec guide to freedom and joy: The teachings of don Miguel Ruiz.* Tulsa, OK: Council Oaks Books.

Neylan, T. (2007). How do you sleep? A conversation with Tom Neylan. University of California, San Francisco, retrieved from http://www.ucsf.edu/news/2007/03/3810/neylan.

Neylan, T., Metzler, T., Best, S., Weiss, D., Fagan, J., Liberman, A., Rogers, C., Vedantham, K., Brunet, A., Lipsey, T., and Marmar, C. (2002). Critical incident exposure and sleep quality in police officers. *Psychosomatic Medicine, 64*(2) 345-352.

Neylan, T., Metzler, T.J., Henn-Haase, C., Blank, Y. Tarasovsky, G., McCaslin, S.E., Lenoci, M., & Marmar, C.R.. (2010). Prior night sleep duration is associated with psychomotor vigilance in a healthy sample of police academy recruits. *Chronobiology International, 27*(7) 1493-1508.

O'Connor, J., & Seymour, J. (2011). *Introducing NLP: Psychological skills for understanding and influencing people.* San Francisco, CA: Conari Press

O'Hara, A.F. & Violanti, J.M. (2009). Police suicide-A web surveillance of national data. *Journal of Emergency Mental Health, 11*(1), 17-23.

Pasca, R., & Wagner, S.L.. (2012). Occupational stress, mental health and satisfaction in the Canadian multicultural workplace. *Social Indicators Research, (109),* 377-393. doi:10.1007/s11205-011-9907-5

Peterson, C. & Seligman, M.E.P. (2004).*Character strength and virtues: A handbook and classification.* Oxford, UK: Oxford University Press.

Pietrzak, R.H., Johnson, D.C., Goldstein, M.B., Malley, J.C., & Southwick, S.M. (2009). Psychological resilience and postdeployment social support protect against traumatic stress and depressive symptoms in soldiers returning from Operations Enduring Freedom and Iraqi Freedom. *Depression and Anxiety, 26*(8), 745-751. doi: 10.1002/da.20558

Pinker, S. (2011). *The better angels of our nature: Why violence has declined.* New York, NY: Penguin Books.

Ruiz, Don Miguel (1997).*The four agreements: A practical guide to personal wisdom.* A Toltec Wisdom Book. San Rafael, CA: Amber-Allen Publishing.

Salo, I. & Allwood, C.M. (2011). Decision-making styles, stress and gender among investigators. *Policing: An International Journal of Police Strategies & Management, 34*(1), 97-119. doi: 10.1108/13639511111106632

Seligman, M.E.P. (2003). *Authentic happiness: Using the new positive psychology to realize your potential for lasting fulfillment.* New York, NY: Free Press, Simon & Schuster.

Seligman, M.E.P. (2011). *Flourish: A visionary new understanding of happiness and well-being.* New York, NY: Free Press, Simon & Schuster.

Seligman, M.E.P. (2011). What is well-being? *Newsletter,* retrieved from www.authentichappiness.sas.upenn.edu/newsletter.aspx?id=1533

Senjo, S.R., & Dhungana, K. (2009). A field data examination of policy constructs related to fatigue conditions in law enforcement personnel. *Police Quarterly,12*(2), 123-136. doi:10.1177/1098611109332420

Shane, J.M. (2010). Organizational stressors and police performance. *Journal of Criminal Justice, 38*(4)807-818. doi: 10.1016/jcrimju2010.05.008

Shapiro, S.L., Astin, J.A., Bishop ,S.R., &Cordova, M. (2005 ). Mindfulness-based stress reduction for health care professionals: Results from a randomized trial. *International Journal of Stress Management, 12*(2) , 164-176.

Siegel, D. J. (2010). *Mindsight: The new science of personal transformation.* New York, NY: Random House.

Speca, R., Carlson, L.E., Goodey, E. & Angen, M.(2000). A randomized, wait-list controlled clinical trial: The effect of a mindfulness meditation-based stress reduction program on mood and symptoms of stress in cancer outpatients. *Psychosomatic Medicine Journal of Biobehavioral Medicine, 62*(5), 613-622.

Spoormaker, V.I., & Montgomery, P. (2008) Disturbed sleep in post-traumatic stress disorder: Secondary symptom or core feature? *Sleep Medicine Reviews, 12*(3), 169-184. doi: 10.1016/j.smrv.2007.08.008

Tanielan, T. (2011). Bridging the gaps in treating veterans with post-deployment mental health problems. *Academy Health.* Rand

Tawny, M. (2008). Integrity testing…The selection tool of the future. *Law & Order, 56*(12), 34-38.

Taylor, S.E., Klein, L.C., Lewis, B.P., Gruenewald, T.L., Gurung, R.A.R., & Updegraff, J.A. (2000). Biobehavioral responses to stress in females: Tend-and-befriend, not fight-or-flight. *Psychological Review, 107*(3) 411-429.

Taylor, S E., Burklund, L.J., Eisenberger, N.I., Lehman, B.J., Hilmert, C.J., & Lieberman, M. D. (2008). Neural bases of moderation of cortisol stress responses by psychosocial resources. *Journal of Personality and Social Psychology, 95*(1), 197-211. doi: 10.1037/0022-3514.95.1.197

University. (2013). *What is Ayurveda?* Integrative Medicine Center, University of Maryland. Retrieved from www. umm.edu/altmed/articles/ayurveda-000348.htm

Vaillant, D. (2003). *Sounds of reform : Progressivism and music in Chicago, 1873-1935.* Chapel Hill, NC: University of North Carolina Press.

Vila, B. (2006). Impact of long work hours on police officers and the communities they serve. *American Journal of Industrial Medicine, 49*(11), 972-980. doi: 10.1002/ajim.20333

Vila, B.J., Kenney, D.J., Morrison, G.B., & Reuland, M. *(*2000*).* Evaluating the effects of fatigue on police patrol officers: Final report. Washington, DC: Police Executive Research

Violanti, J.M., (n.d.). A resilient police organization makes the difference. *The Jimston Journal.* Retrieved from www.jimstonjournal.com/id147.html.

Violanti, J.M. (n.d.). Stress, a police health problem. *The Jimston Journal.* Retrieved from www.jimstonjournal.com/id128.html

Violanti, J.M. (n.d.). The disabled police officer – gone and forgotten. The *Jimston Journal.* Retrieved from http://jimsonjournal.com/id141.html.

Violanti, J.M. (2010) Police suicide: A national comparison with fire-fighter and military personnel. *Policing: An International Journal of Police Strategies & Management, 33*(2) 270-286.
doi:    10.1108/13639511011044885

Violanti, J.M.., Fekedulegn, D., Hartley, T.A., Andrew, M.E., Charles, L.E., Mnatsakanova, A., & Burchfiel, C.M. (2006). Police trauma and cardiovascular disease: Association between PTSD symptoms and metabolic syndrome. *International Journal of Emergency Mental Health, 8*(4):227-37.

Violanti, J.M., Fekedulegn, D., Andrew, M.E., Charles, L.E., Hartley, T., & Burchfiel, C.M. (2007). Adiposity and depressive symptoms in police officers. *Annals of Epidemiology, 17*(9), 734. doi:10.1016/j.annepidem.2007.07.037

Violanti, J.M., Burchfiel, C.M, Hartley, T.A., Mnatsakanova, A., Fekedulegn, D., Andrew, M.E., Charles, L.E., &. Vila, B.J. (2009). Atypical work hours and metabolic syndrome among police officers. *Environmental & Occupational Health, 64*(3), 194-201. doi: 10.1080/19338240903241259

Violanti, J.M., Fekedulegn, D., Andrew, M.E., Charles, L.E., Hartley, T.A., Vila, B., and Burchfiel, C.M. (2012). Shift work and the incidence of injury among police officers. *American Journal of Industrial Medicine. Online:* doi: 10.1002/ajim.22007.

Wang, J.J., Korczykowski, M., Rao, H., Fan, Y., Pluta, J., Gur, R.C., McEwen, B.S.,& Detre, J.A. (2007) Gender difference in neural responses to psychological stress. *Social Cognitive &Affective Neuroscience 2*(3): 227-239.

Wang, Z., Inslicht, S.S., Metzler, T.J., Henne-Haase, C., McCaslin, S.E., Tong, H., Neylan, T.C., & Marmar, C.R. (2010). A prospective study of predictors of depression symptoms in police. *Psychiatry Research, 175*(3), 211-216. doi: 10.1016/j.psychres.2008.11.010

Weil, A. (2011). *Spontaneous happiness.* New York, NY: Little, Brown.

Weiss, D.S., & Marmar, C.R. (1997). The Impact of Event Scale-Revised. In J.P. Wilson & T.M. Keane (Eds.), *Assessing Psychological Trauma and PTSD* (pp.399-411). New York, NY: Guilford.

Wertheim, P.A. (1998). Integrity assurance: Policies and procedures to prevent fabrication of latent print evidence. *Journal of Forensic Identification, 48*(4), 431-431.

Westen, P.K. (2010). Answer self-incriminating questions or be fired. *American Journal of Criminal Law, 37*(2), 97-162.

Witteveen, A.B., Van der Ploeg, E., Bramsen, I., Huizink, A.C., Slottje, P., Smid, T., & Van der Ploeg, H.M. (2006). Dimensionality of the posttraumatic stress response among police officers and fire fighters: An evaluation of two self-report scales. *Psychiatry Research,* 41(2):213-28.

Witteveen, A.B, Huizink , A.C., Slottje, P., Bramsen, I., Smid, T., & van der Ploeg, H..M. (2010). Associations of cortisol with posttraumatic stress symptoms and negative life events: A study of police officers and firefighters. *Psychoneuroendocrinology 35*(7), 1113-1118.

Worthen, M. D. & Moering, R.G. (2011). A practical guide to conducting VA compensation and pension exams for PTSD and other mental disorders. *Psychological Injury and the Law,* (4), 3-4,187-216. doi:10.1007/s12207-011-9115-2

Yuan, C., Wang, Z. , Inslicht, S.S., McCaslin, S.E., Metzler, T.J.,  Henn-Haase, C. , Apfel, B.A., Tong, H., Neylan, T.C.,  Fang, Y., & Marmar, C.R.. (2011). Protective factors for posttraumatic stress disorder symptoms in a prospective study of police officers. *Psychiatry Research, 188*(1), 45-50. doi: 10.1016/j.psychres.2010.10.034

Zeidan, F.,  Martucci, K.T., Kraft, R.A., Gordon, N.S., Hafflie, J.G., & Coghill, R.(2011). Brain mechanisms supporting the modulation of pain by mindfulness meditation. *Journal of Neuroscience, 31*(14) 5540-5548. doi: 10.1523/JNEUROSCI.5791-10.2011

# Appendix I — Definitions

Definitions are frequently modified to reflect new information as researchers continue to explore the complexity of good health and the complexity of afflictions resulting from exposure and reaction to high-stress environments. The following definitions are not intended to be diagnostic tools; they are offered as guidelines throughout this work with the hope that prevention of stress-related illnesses may be heightened by mindful attention. Readers are encouraged to pursue professional advice and diagnosis in cases where illness may be related to high-stress situations.

*Acute Stress Disorder (ASD)* symptoms may arise shortly after an individual experiences an event perceived as an extreme threat. An intense sense of helplessness or fear may accompany disorientation, impaired consciousness, numbing, narrowing of attention, impaired judgment, and apparent inability to understand various stimuli. The physiological aspects of ASD relate to the sympathetic nervous system which releases adrenaline and noradrenaline at the onset of stress and facilitates physical reactions. Duration of the response symptoms vary widely, and various therapies, including cognitive behavioral therapy, may be beneficial in treating psychological aspects of ASD.

*Amygdala* is a small, almond-shaped part of the brain located in the temporal lobes and associated with emotions and aggression. As part of the limbic system, the amygdala functions to control the secretion of hormones, arousal, fear responses, and the formation of emotional memories.

*Anxiety* is characterized by disquieting feelings of dread, worry, and general uneasiness. It may be considered a normal reaction to stressor(s), but it can occur without an obvious triggering event and may be considered a disorder when symptoms are prolonged and excessive, involving sleep, emotional, cognitive, and behavioral components. Immune and digestive functions may be inhibited, and the condition may involve heart palpitations, fatigue, muscle weakness, nausea, headaches, and increased blood pressure and heart rate.

*Anxiety Sensitivity (AS)* is characterized by an individual's inclination to fear anxiety-related symptoms such as headache, increased heart rate, sweating, or muscle tension An individual suffering anxiety sensitivity may believe that there are negative physical, social, or mental outcomes associated with the symptoms. The condition is sometimes referred to as "fear of fear".

*Comprehensive Soldier Fitness (CSF)* is a long-term assessment and development program pursued by the US Army to utilize positive psychology to build resilience and enhance the performance of soldiers, civilian personnel, and family members (http://csf.army.mil/).

*Cortisol* is the major hormone produced by the adrenal cortex to maintain blood pressure and regulate carbohydrate metabolism and the immune system. Its normal pattern is to become elevated as a person wakes from sleep, to level off throughout the day, and to decrease at night. Under conditions of extreme stress, however, the pattern may be seriously disrupted. The response becomes maladaptive when the body's reaction is not healthfully controlled by normal regulatory mechanisms.

*EmWave* is an easy-to-use monitoring and training device developed by the Institute of HeartMath to help transform stress reactions, improve wellness, and enhance personal growth. See page 39 for a thorough discussion of emWave technology and the Institute.

*Health.* Dr. Andrew Weil, a co-developer of and strong spokesman for integrative medicine, describes health as "A dynamic condition of wholeness and balance that allows us to move through life and not succumb to malfunctions of our own physiology or suffer harm from all the potentially damaging influences we encounter" (Weil, 2011, p.6).

*Hyperarousal* describes an aggregate of psychological and physiological symptoms that result from high levels of anxiety. They include irritability, anger outbursts, being easily startled, reduced pain tolerance, insomnia, having difficulty concentrating, and feeling constantly vigilant against unspecified danger.

*Hypervigilance* is an intensified state of sensory sensitivity resulting in exaggerated behaviors. Individuals who experience hypervigilance may be preoccupied with scanning environments for threats, and the hypervigilant state may be accompanied by high-level anxiety, abnormal arousal responses, and sleep disorders. Exhaustion frequently accompanies hypervigilant states.

*Impact of Event Scale (IES) and Revised Scale (IES-R)* are screening tools developed in 1979 by Harowitz, Wilner, and Alvarez (IES) and modified in 1997 by Weiss and Marmar (IES-R). Both IES and the revised version are subjective tests intended to identify the impact of traumatic events experienced by individuals.

*Metabolic Syndrome* is an aggregation of factors that heighten the risk for coronary artery disease, stroke, and type-2 diabetes. All of the risks are related to obesity, and the risk factors have also been associated with psychological conditions. Individuals suffering from metabolic syndrome typically have excess weight around their waists (a useful preliminary screening tool), and they may also experience excess blood clotting and low levels of inflammation throughout the body.

*NEO Five-Factor Personality Inventory* is a psychological personality inventory used with adult men and women who do not exhibit overt psychopathology. The five factors examined are extraversion, agreeableness, conscientiousness, neuroticism, and openness to experience. The assessment tool was developed by Paul T.

Costa, Jr. and Robert R. McCrae, and an article by McCrae and O.P. John (1992) provides an introduction to the model and its applications.

**Obesity (Adiposity)** is a condition in which the body has stored excess fat, which increases the likelihood of adverse health issues including reduced life expectancy, heart disease, type 2 diabetes, sleep apnea, osteoarthritis, and some types of cancer. Obesity is not defined in terms of body weight but in terms of the amount of body fat in an individual's adipose tissue – connective tissue whose cells normally function to store energy and to cushion and insulate the body. *Adiposity* is the medical term for obesity.

**Peritraumatic incidents** are events occurring around the time of trauma.

**Post Traumatic Stress Disorder (PTSD).** The language path from "battle fatigue" to PTSD has been bumpy, ornate, and oft-times controversial. Since 1954, the American Psychiatric Association has published and updated the manual *Diagnostic and Statistical Manual of Mental Disorders* (DSM) to provide researchers, clinicians, pharmaceutical and insurance companies, and policy and regulation agencies with common language and criteria for classifying mental disorders. The manual is a standard in the United States while the *International Classification of Diseases*, produced by the World Health Organization, is more frequently used in Europe and throughout other parts of the world. The DSM manual has undergone five revisions, the most recent in 2000 (DSM-IV-TR). An update is scheduled for 2013. The DSM diagnostic criteria for PTSD are shown in the chart on page 12.

**Serotonin** is a hormone found in the human pineal gland, brain, blood serum, and gastric mucous membranes. It acts as a chemical messenger to transmit signals between nerve cells and is active in inhibition of gastric secretion, stimulation of smooth muscles, and production of vasoconstriction, and regulation of cyclic body processes. In the central nervous system, serotonin regulates mood, appetite, sleep, memory, and learning; it is associated with feelings of happiness and decreased anxiety. Changes in the serotonin levels in the brain can alter individuals' moods.

www.ingramcontent.com/pod-product-compliance
Lightning Source LLC
Chambersburg PA
CBHW082136290526
45794CB00008B/3056